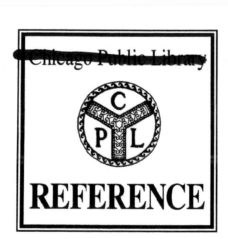

An Atlas of
ORTHOPEDIC SURGERY
A Guide to Management and Practice

THE ENCYCLOPEDIA OF VISUAL MEDICINE SERIES

An Atlas of
ORTHOPEDIC SURGERY
A Guide to Management and Practice

Edward V. Craig, MD

Attending Orthopedic Surgery
The Hospital for Special Surgery
New York, NY, USA

Beth E. Shubin Stein, MD

Assistant Attending Orthopedic Surgery
The Hospital for Special Surgery
New York, NY, USA

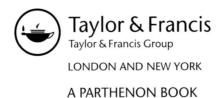

Taylor & Francis
Taylor & Francis Group

LONDON AND NEW YORK

A PARTHENON BOOK

First published in the United Kingdom in 2004
by Taylor & Francis,
an imprint of the Taylor & Francis Group,
11 New Fetter Lane,
London EC4P 4EE

Tel.:   +44 (0) 20 7583 9855
Fax.:   +44 (0) 20 7842 2298
Website: www.tandf.co.uk

British Library Cataloguing in Publication Data

Data available on application

Library of Congress Cataloging-in-Publication Data

Data available on application

ISBN 1-84214-185-6

Distributed in North and South America by

Taylor & Francis
2000 NW Corporate Blvd
Boca Raton, FL 33431, USA

Within Continental USA
Tel.: 800 272 7737; Fax.: 800 374 3401
Outside Continental USA
Tel.: 561 994 0555; Fax.: 561 361 6018
E-mail: orders@crcpress.com

Distributed in the rest of the world by
Thomson Publishing Services
Cheriton House
North Way
Andover, Hampshire SP10 5BE, UK
Tel.: +44 (0) 1264 332424
E-mail: salesorder.tandf@thomsonpublishingservices.co.uk

Composition by Parthenon Publishing
Printed and bound by T.G. Hostench, S.A., Spain

Contents

Preface

We hope that this Atlas will be useful as a reference guide to the most common disorders of Orthopedic Surgery for the clinician as well as for those who are training for a career in Orthopedics.

The field of Orthopedics is vast and certainly cannot be covered in its entirety in one Atlas. However, we have hopefully succeeded in selecting the most common and most clinically relevant topics. The goal of this Atlas is to illustrate a wide range of orthopedic conditions that are representative of the field and its subspecialties.

We would like to thank the doctors who so graciously contributed both their clinical experience and their library of pictures which were of great assistance in putting together this Atlas:

Dr Michael Vitale, Pediatric Orthopedics; Drs Scott Wolfe and Pamela Sherman, Hand and Wrist; Dr Andrew Elliott, Foot and Ankle; and Dr Andrew Sama, Spine; and Dr Christopher S. Ahmad, Knee and Elbow.

Beth E. Shubin Stein, MD
Edward V. Craig, MD

Chapter 1

The hand and wrist

Hand surgery is a subspecialty that is frequently an area for additional training beyond the general training in one's primary specialty (e.g. orthopedic surgery or plastic surgery). Most hand problems are seen initially by non-specialists and so it is important for all physicians to have a general knowledge about the field so that they can decide when to refer a patient to a hand surgeon.

ANATOMY

The wrist or carpus is the junction of the distal radius and ulna with the hand. The carpal bones include the scaphoid, lunate, triquetrum, pisiform, trapezium, trapezoid, capitate and hamate. The carpal bones are involved in a multitude of articulations. These bones connect the distal radius and ulna to the metacarpals and phalangeal bones of the fingers. A large section of this chapter is devoted to the scaphoid in particular. Of the carpal bones, the scaphoid is the most susceptible to fracture and also to complications after fracture due to its unique blood supply. Carpal stability is increased by its numerous ligamentous connections, and injury to these ligaments often leads to instability and eventual arthritis.

The carpal metacarpal joints connect the wrist to the fingers and are often affected by systemic conditions such as lupus, rheumatoid arthritis and gout. The trapezium–metacarpal joint (the basalar joint of the thumb), in particular, is a common source of pain (more often in women) due to osteoarthritis. This debilitating condition causes tremendous pain and stiffness and can significantly limit the use of the thumb in daily activities such as opening jars, buttoning a shirt and even brushing one's teeth. There are five metacarpal bones that connect to the phalanges. The thumb has only proximal and distal phalanges, whereas the other four fingers are composed of proximal, middle and distal phalanges. The muscles of the forearm cross the wrist and insert as tendons, allowing wrist and finger motion.

The dorsum of the wrist is divided into six extensor compartments. The first dorsal compartment contains the extensor pollicis brevis and the abductor pollicis longus to the thumb. This compartment is often a site of acute inflammation called DeQuervain's tenosynovitis. The second compartment contains the extensor carpi radialis brevis and longus. The third compartment contains the extensor pollicis longus, the fourth compartment the extensor digitorum communis and extensor indicis, the fifth the extensor digiti minimi (to the little finger) and the sixth compartment the extensor carpi ulnaris.

The carpal tunnel is located on the volar aspect of the wrist. The roof of the carpal tunnel is the transverse carpal ligament and this is the structure that is released during carpal tunnel surgery. The carpal canal contains the median nerve as well as the tendons of the flexor digitorum profundus, flexor digitorum superficialis and flexor pollicis longus.

HISTORY AND PHYSICAL EXAMINATION

Pathological conditions of the hand can be divided into several categories: congenital, acquired, traumatic, and inflammatory. It is important to take a history specific to the type of problem. For example, if a patient is being evaluated for a congenital hand deformity, it is important to find out about the rest of the family members and the pregnancy. If the patient was involved in an accident, the physician should find out specific details of the environment in which the accident or trauma occurred. Was it on a farm or at home in the kitchen? All of these details can help to lead the clinician to the diagnosis and also aid in formulating the treatment. It is important to find out which hand is dominant and what the patient does for a living (e.g manual laborer vs. desk job). If the patient describes an insidious onset, then the physician should question the longevity of the symptoms, symptom progression, functional limitations, and what makes the pain better or worse.

Inspection of the upper extremities includes documentation of any skin lesions, color changes or asymmetries between the affected and contralateral limbs and this is frequently the primary diagnositic modality in such cases as congenital hand lesions or Dupuytren's contractures. Systemic conditions, such as psoriasis, Raynaud's, rheumatoid arthritis or scleroderma, frequently have characteristic hand manifestations. Complete upper extremity examination should be systematic, beginning with the shoulders and cervical spine. The range of motion of the shoulders, elbows, forearm rotation, wrist and fingers are all recorded. Motor strength testing and a careful peripheral neurological examination of the radial, median and ulnar nerves are critical, along with a check of the vascular system.

DIAGNOSTIC STUDIES

Plain radiographs can be valuable in cases of trauma or congenital deformities. However, there are many small bones in the wrist and a fracture is often difficult to detect. Computed tomography (CT) scanning can be helpful in evaluating difficult fractures of the carpal bones. Bone scanning or magnetic resonance imaging (MRI) are excellent modalities to use when looking for an occult fracture such as may occur in the scaphoid. MRI is also a useful tool in evaluating soft tissue injuries to the hand. Though frank tendon ruptures are often easily diagnosed from the history and physical examination, the diagnosis of some injuries such as triangular–fibrocartilage complex injuries and scapholunate disruptions may be better evaluated with the use of MRI.

DISORDERS

The most common disorders of the hand and wrist are illustrated in Figures 1–31.

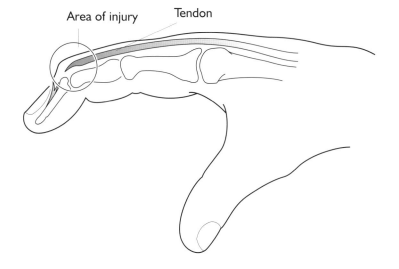

Area of injury   Tendon

Figure 1   Diagram illustrating the area of the injury in a mallet finger. A mallet injury is an avulsion of the terminal extensor tendon as it inserts onto the proximal aspect of the distal phalanx on the dorsal surface

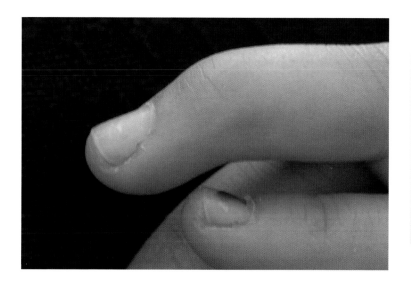

Figure 2   Clinical photograph of a patient who sustained a mallet injury. Mallet injuries can be either bony (an avulsion fracture of the distal phalanx) or purely soft tissue. In cases where the injury is to soft tissue, or the fracture fragment is small, treatment involves extension splinting for 6 weeks full-time. The chronic mallet finger can be treated as a fresh injury for up to 4 weeks with good results

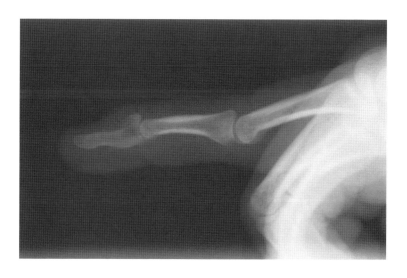

Figure 3   Lateral radiograph of a large bony mallet with the fracture fragment comprising about 40% of the joint surface; the distal interphalangeal joint is volarly subluxed. This requires reduction of the fragment with k-wire fixation

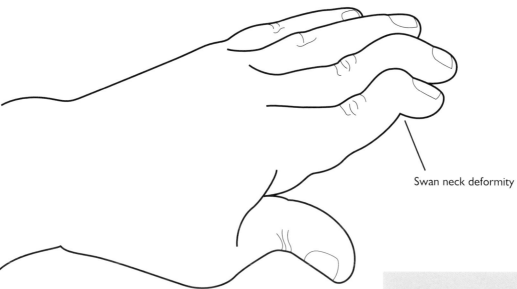

Swan neck deformity

a

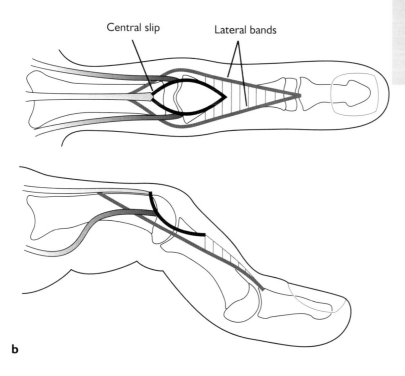

Central slip   Lateral bands

b

Figure 4 Diagrams illustrating several other tendon disorders of the hand. The swan neck (a) deformity is characterized by hyperextension of the proximal interphalangeal joint and flexion of the distal interphalangeal joint. It is usually caused by an uneven pull of the tendons at the proximal interphalangeal joint and volar plate laxity or injury. The boutonniere deformity (b) is characterized by the exactly opposite posture, with flexion at the proximal interphalangeal joint and resultant hyperextension of the distal interphalangeal joint. The deformity is caused by central slip attenuation or rupture and volar subluxation of the lateral bands

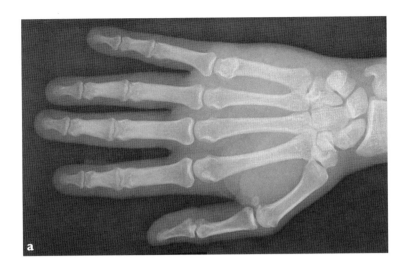

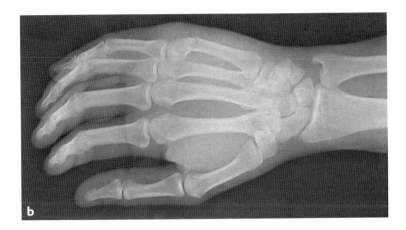

Figure 5 Anteroposterior (a) and oblique (b) radiographs of a young male who was in a fight and sustained this boxer's fracture of the 5th metacarpal neck. These fractures can usually be treated non-operatively with cast immobilization. However, this patient had significant angulation at the neck and a rotational deformity clinically that led the surgeon to elect a closed reduction and pinning as seen in (c). The patient went on to heal the fracture uneventfully

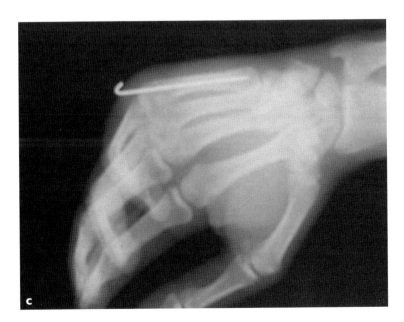

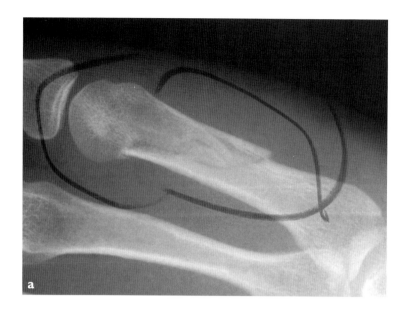

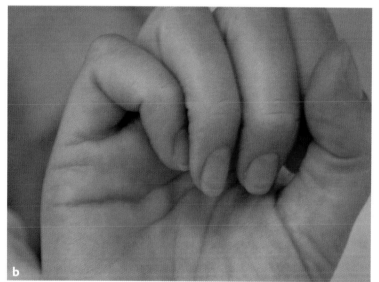

Figure 6 Metacarpal shaft fractures can usually be treated with cast immobilization. However, if significant comminution exists or there is a clinical rotatory deformity, then open reduction with internal fixation is indicated. This patient sustained a comminuted midshaft 5th metacarpal fracture with rotational deformity (a and b) and underwent open reduction with internal fixation, as shown in (c), with good results

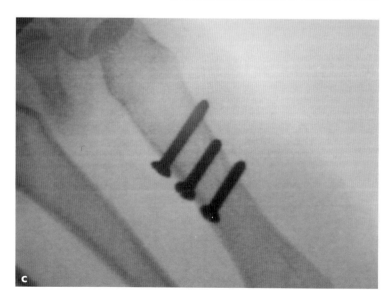

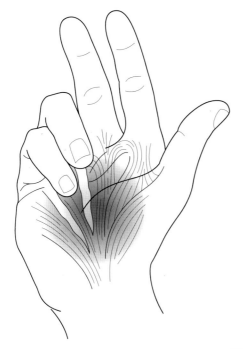

a

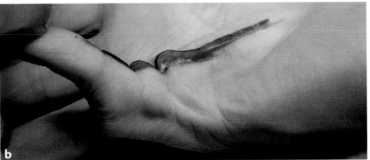

b

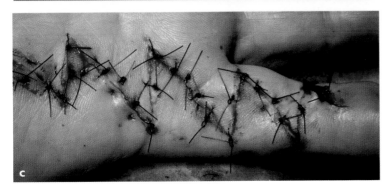

c

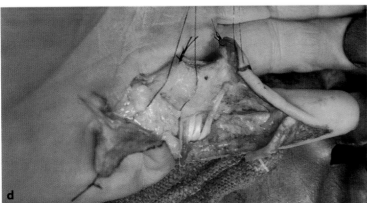

d

Figure 7 Dupuytren's contracture (a) is a disease characterized by progressive interphalangeal contractures caused by fascial tightening. The disease is more prevalent in northern Europeans and males and generally occurs after the 4th decade. The disease is associated with alcoholism, diabetes, epilepsy and chronic pulmonary disease. The disease causes a change in the normal fascial bands to the diseased cords, leading to the contractures. In addition, these cords put the neurovascular bundle at risk by displacing it volarly and proximally. Stretching exercises have not proven useful; cortisone injections may slow the progression of cord formation. Ultimately, surgical intervention is indicated when either the metacarpalphalangeal or proximal interphalangeal contractures are greater than 30° (b–d)

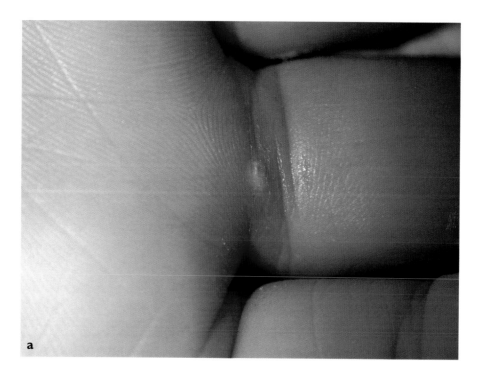

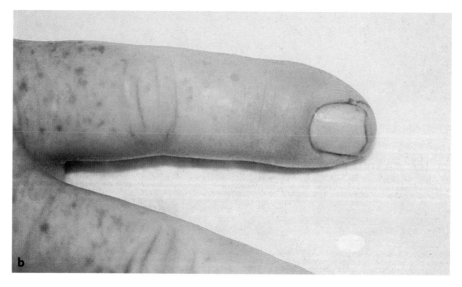

Figure 8   Infections can progress and spread rapidly due to the abundance of communicating spaces in the hand. It is important to determine the origin or source of infection based on history because certain organisms are more likely, depending on where and how the injury occurred. For example, a human bite is a serious source of infection (a) and, although *Staphylococcus aureus* and *Streptococcus* are the most likely pathogens, one must be aware of the potential for infection with *Eikenella corrodens* and cover with the appropriate antibiotics after a complete irrigation and debridement. An infection in or around the nail-fold is called paronychia (b),

Continued

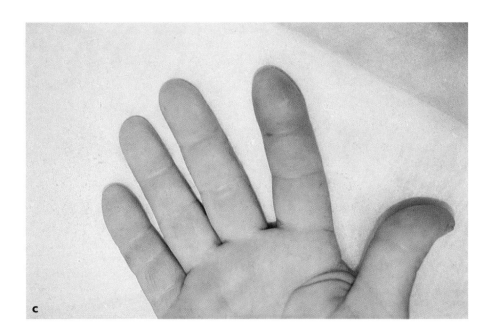

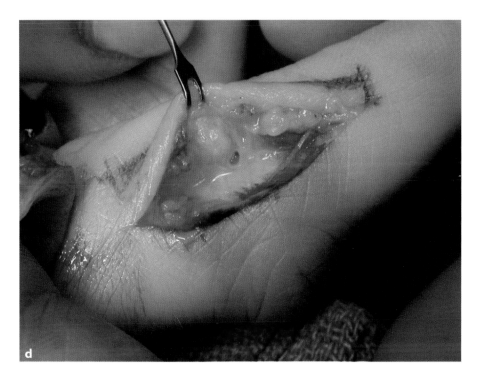

Figure 8 *continued* an infection of the pulp of the finger tip is called a felon (c), and infection in the tendon sheath of the finger is called suppurative flexor tenosynovitis.

The cardinal signs of a flexor sheath infection are called the Kanavel signs. These are swelling of the entire finger, flexed posture of the finger, and pain with passive extension and tenderness over the flexor sheath. If the infections are diagnosed early, most are treated adequately with intravenous antibiotics. However, copious irrigation and debridement are required (d) if the infection progresses and/or is unresponsive to the choice of antibiotics

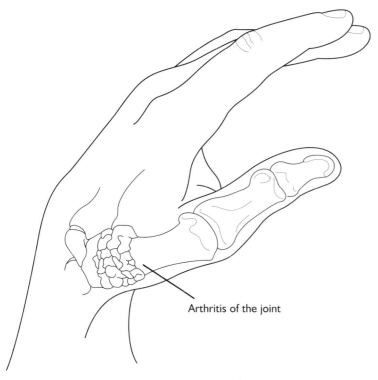

Arthritis of the joint

Figure 9 Diagram of an arthritic basalar joint of the thumb. The carpometacarpal joint of the thumb is an extremely important joint for functions such as the pinch and grasp. Women tend to have a higher incidence of basalar joint osteoarthritis and the reasons for this are currently under investigation. When advanced, arthritis of this joint can significantly limit one's ability to perform activities of daily living (e.g. brushing teeth, combing hair and opening jars)

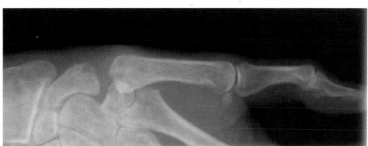

Figure 10 Anteroposterior radiograph of a patient who underwent a basilar joint arthroplasty for advanced carpometacarpal arthritis. Excision of the trapezium and interposition arthroplasty with a soft tissue graft (e.g. palmaris tendon) alleviate the pain and significantly improve motion at this joint. However, there is a decrease in pinch strength in the long term

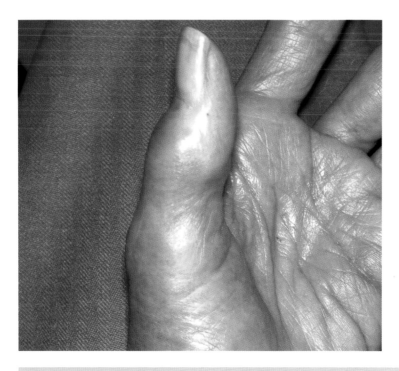

Figure 11 Clinical photograph of a patient 4 weeks after a basilar joint arthroplasty with improved ability to abduct the thumb

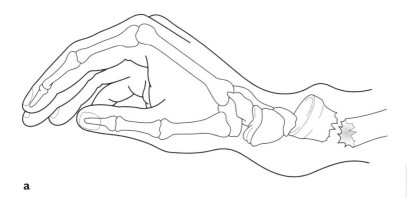

a

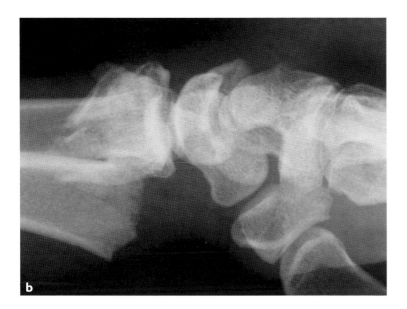

b

Figure 12 Diagram (a) and lateral radiograph (b) of a distal radius fracture, the so-called Colles fracture. The mechanism of injury is a fall onto an outstretched hand, causing dorsal displacement of the distal fracture fragment. If the fracture is not intra-articular and not significantly comminuted, then most will do well with closed reduction and casting

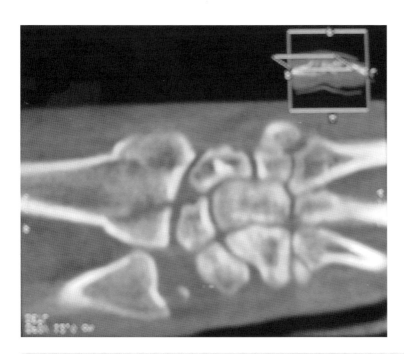

Figure 13 Pre-operative CT scans can often be helpful if there is a comminuted intra-articular fracture. Radiographs are often difficult to read due to the comminution, making fracture classification and pre-operative planning problematic

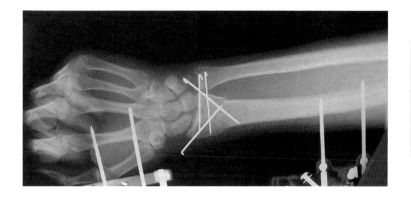

Figure 14 Anteroposterior radiograph of the fracture postoperatively. An external fixator was applied to maintain length and then the intra-articular fragments were reduced and pinned

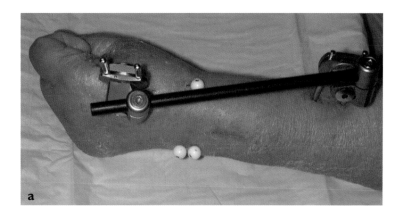

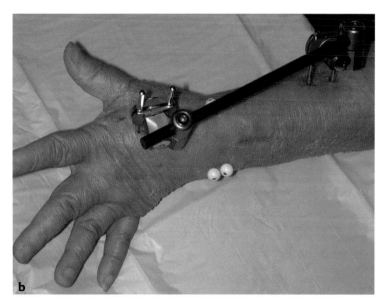

Figure 15 Clinical photographs (a and b) showing a patient after placement of an external fixator. The surgeon should be careful not to over distract the wrist, thus making the full range of motion of the hand difficult. Pin tract infections are a problem when dealing with external fixators and the patients should be instructed on how to clean the pin sites daily

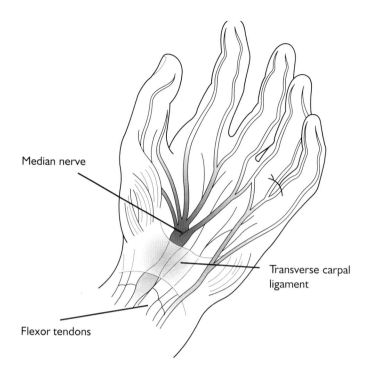

Median nerve

Transverse carpal ligament

Flexor tendons

Figure 16 Diagram of the carpal tunnel illustrating the median nerve passing under the transverse carpal ligament. Swelling in this tunnel (due to trauma or synovitis) can increase the pressure on the nerve, causing symptoms of numbness and pain

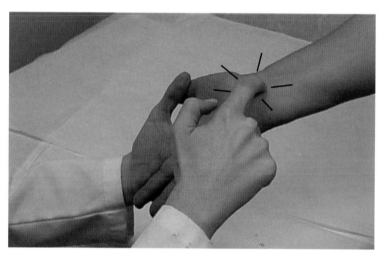

Figure 17 The Tinel sign is elicited by tapping lightly over the carpal tunnel and reproducing the patient's symptoms of pain and/or tingling

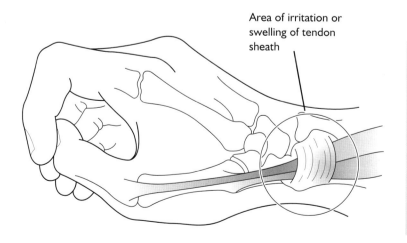

Area of irritation or swelling of tendon sheath

Figure 18 Diagram illustrating the pathology associated with stenosing tenosynovitis of the first dorsal compartment (DeQuervain's tenosynovitis). The pathogenesis is inflammation of the tenosynovium within the first dorsal compartment. The extensor pollicis brevis and the abductor pollicis longus run through this compartment, making use of the thumb, in this condition, very painful

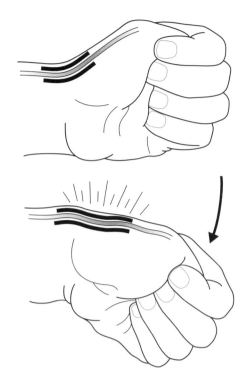

a

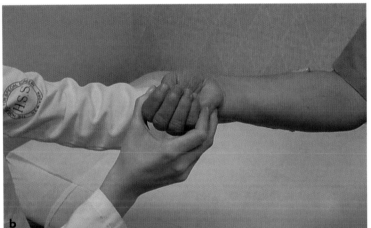

b

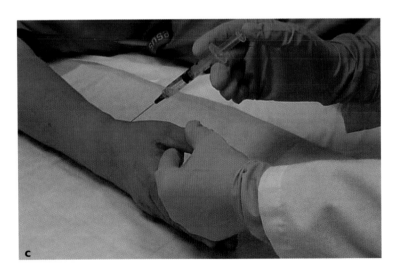

c

Figure 19 Finkelstein's test is a provocative maneuver designed to elicit pain in patients with DeQuervain's tenosynovitis (a). The ipsilateral thumb is grasped within a clenched fist and the fist is then ulnarly deviated by either the patient or the physician (b). Reproduction of the same pain radiating proximally within the tendon sheath is considered a positive test. Treatment for this tenosynovitis consists of thumb spica splinting to reduce motion, anti-inflammatory medication and/or cortisone injections into the sheath (c). Those cases that do not respond to the treatments described may need to undergo surgery to release the first dorsal compartment. Complications associated with this surgery include injury to the sensory branch of the radial nerve or failure to decompress the extensor pollicis brevis, which sometimes lies in a separate compartment

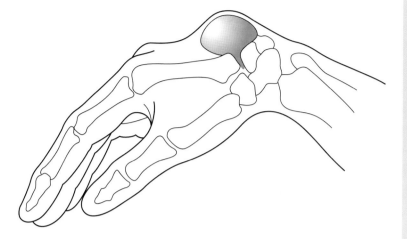

Figure 20 Ganglion cysts of the wrist are most commonly located on the dorsal aspect of the wrist. The dorsal cysts usually arise from the scapholunate joint. When seen on the volar aspect of the wrist, the cysts are usually found to arise from the scaphotrapezial joints. The cyst fluid is a gelatinous material that can be aspirated, but recurrences are high with this technique. Surgical excision, when properly performed to include the stalk from the joint capsule, has a recurrence rate of about 10%

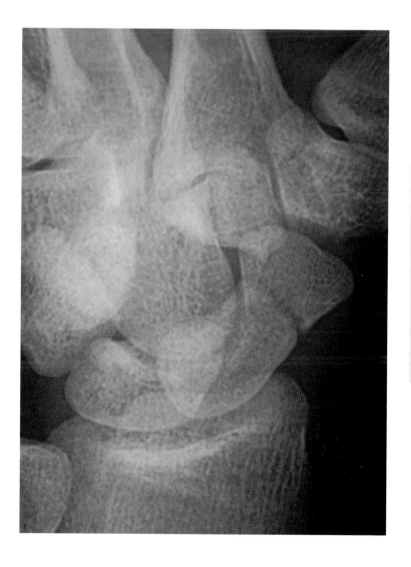

Figure 21 Anteroposterior radiograph of a displaced scaphoid fracture. Scaphoid fractures are sometimes not seen on the initial radiographs. If a scaphoid fracture is suspected clinically (snuff-box tenderness), the patient should be immobilized in a thumb spica cast and the radiographs repeated in 2 weeks (when some fracture resorption makes visualization easier). Alternatively, a bone scan, CT or MRI can be obtained to make the diagnosis

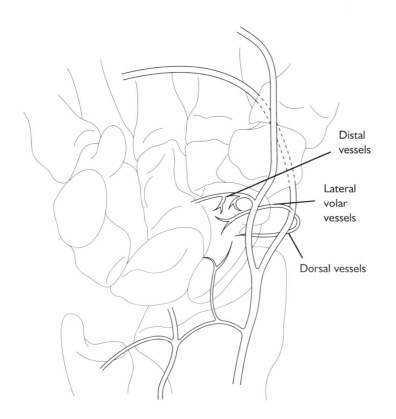

Distal vessels

Lateral volar vessels

Dorsal vessels

Figure 22 Diagram illustrating the blood supply to the scaphoid. This bone receives its major blood supply distally, making avascular necrosis and non-union much more likely than in other bones that have a proximal-to-distal blood supply

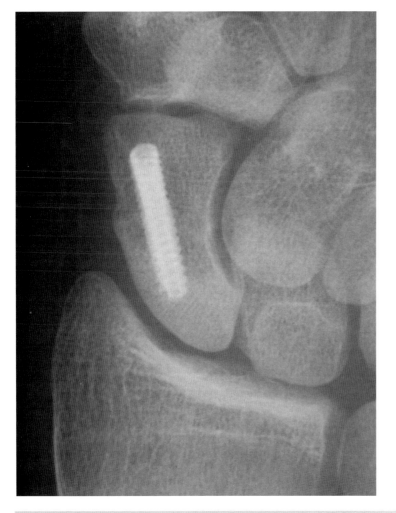

Figure 23 Scaphoid fractures that are displaced and fractures that have gone on to non-union should be surgically treated. This anteroposterior radiograph demonstrates the surgical reduction and screw fixation. Non-unions are more difficult to treat and can require bone grafting in order to achieve union and avoid avascular necrosis

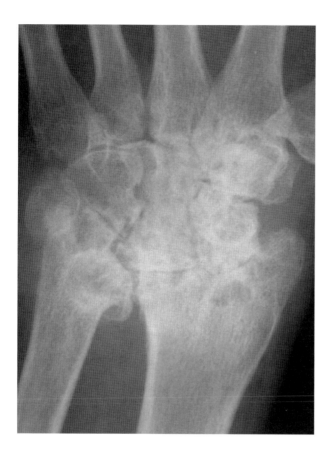

Figure 24 Anteroposterior radiograph of a wrist with advanced degenerative disease

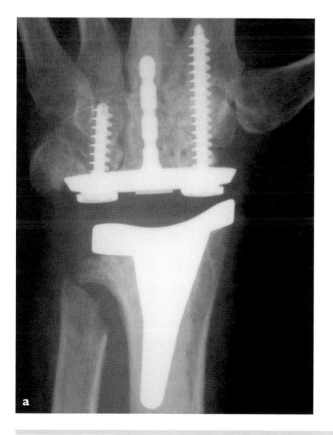

Figures 25 Anteroposterior (a) and lateral (b) postoperative radiographs of a total wrist arthroplasty in a patient with advanced degenerative disease

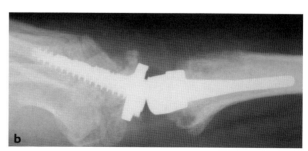

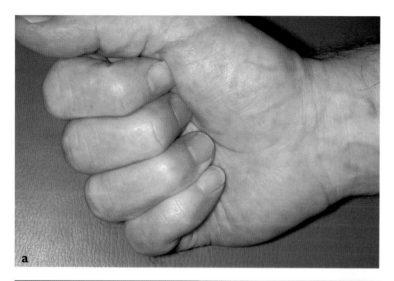

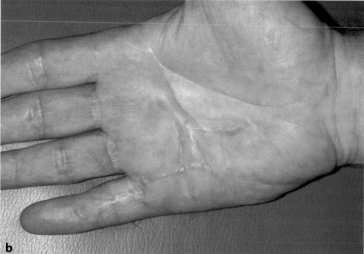

Figure 26 Postoperative clinical photographs of a patient 3 months after a total wrist arthroplasty. The patient had significant relief of his pain, and increased mobility in the hand. Dorsiflexion and plantar flexion vary and are usually related to the patient's pre-operative motion

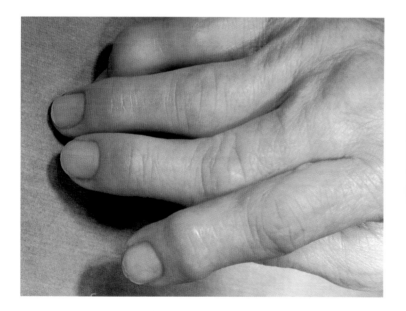

Figure 27 Clinical photograph of a patient with rheumatoid arthritis. The common ulnar deviation of the fingers is well illustrated

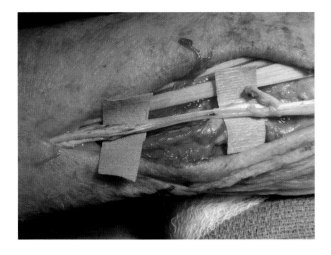

Figure 28 Patients with rheumatoid arthritis often develop characteristic hand and wrist deformities. Wrist instability causes increased pressure in the extensor compartments, which are already affected by the pervasive rheumatoid synovitis. The increased pressure can lead to necrosis, attrition and subsequent rupture of the extensor tendons ('Vaughn-Jackson syndrome'). If this is recognized early, surgical synovectomy can slow the progression of this disease process

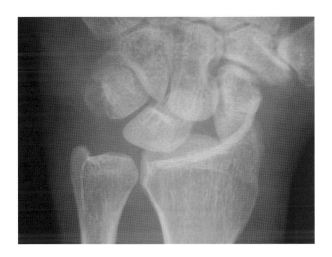

Figure 29 Anteroposterior radiograph of the clenched fist of a patient with an injury to the scapholunate ligament. Note the widened scapholunate gap. Patients with scapholunate ligament disruption and a gap greater than 3 mm on an anteroposterior clenched-fist view (Terry Thomas sign) should have the ligament surgically repaired to prevent progressive carpal instability

Figure 30 Gradient-echo coronal oblique MRI demonstrating a tear in the triangular–fibrocartilage complex (TFCC). All traumatic injuries to the TFCC (not associated with other carpal injuries) are initially treated with immobilization and anti-inflammatory medication. Patients whose symptoms persist are usually treated surgically

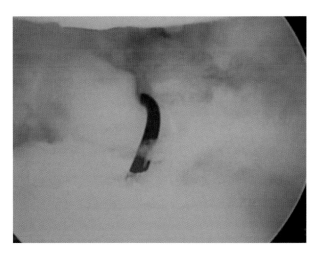

Figure 31 Arthroscopic photograph of a repair of the triangular–fibrocartilage complex. The tear can either be treated with surgical resection or a repair based on its morphology and location

Chapter 2

The elbow

ANATOMY

The bones of the elbow consist of the distal humerus and the proximal radius and ulna. The distal humerus has a lateral column made up of the capitellum, and a corresponding medial side made up of the trochlea. The proximal aspect of the ulna, the olecranon, articulates with the trochlea, and the proximal radial head with the capitellum. The medial (ulnar) and lateral (radial) collateral ligaments provide static restraint to valgus and varus stresses, respectively. The medial collateral ligament is made up of the anterior, posterior and transverse bands. The lateral collateral ligament runs obliquely between the lateral epicondyle and ulna. The annular ligament encircles the radial neck, stabilizing the radiocapitellar articulation. The lateral epicondyle of the humerus serves as the origin of the extensor/supinator mass, and the medial epicondyle is the origin for the flexor/pronator mass.

HISTORY AND PHYSICAL EXAMINATION

Specific questions as to the location and nature of the pain, radiation of the pain, and activities that exacerbate the pain are all important in leading to a diagnosis. Any history of trauma or repetitive activity should also be carefully elicited. Inspection and palpation are the first steps in the physical examination. Inspection should document angular alignment. Normal alignment averages approximately 5° of valgus for men and 10–15° of valgus in women. This carrying angle can be significantly altered in cases of old trauma, especially in the pedi-

atric population. Deformity may also be a clue to tendon injuries such as distal ruptures of the biceps and triceps. The range of motion is checked and compared to that of the opposite side. The normal range of motion is 0–135° and pronation and supination are generally a full 90° in both directions. Bony palpation followed by soft tissue palpation of the ligamentous and tendinous structures provides useful information in establishing the differential diagnosis. Provocative maneuvers are used to test the competence of the ligaments and specific tendon injuries (i.e. extensor carpi radialis brevis in tennis elbow). Motor testing is performed for all the major muscle groups that cross the elbow.

DIAGNOSTIC STUDIES

Plain radiographs (anteroposterior and lateral) are valuable in cases of trauma and to identify loose bodies and can also be helpful in diagnosing degenerative conditions. For soft tissue pathologies, magnetic resonance imaging (MRI) is more useful. In cases of injury to specific structures such as the medial or lateral collateral ligaments, a magnetic resonance arthrogram can often assist to visualize the pathology.

DISORDERS

Disorders of the elbow are illustrated in Figures 32–52.

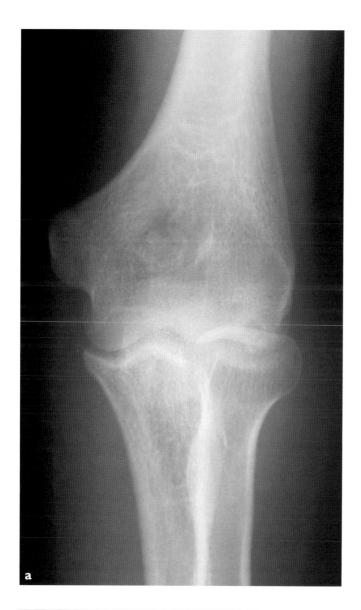

Figure 32 Anteroposterior (a) and lateral (b) radiographs of an elbow with a loose body in the coronoid fossa. The loose body can be seen in shadow on the anteroposterior radiograph, but is better localized on the lateral radiograph. This loose body caused symptoms of catching and an inability to flex the elbow fully in this patient

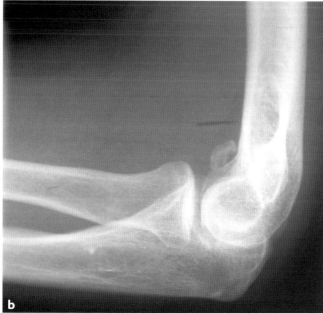

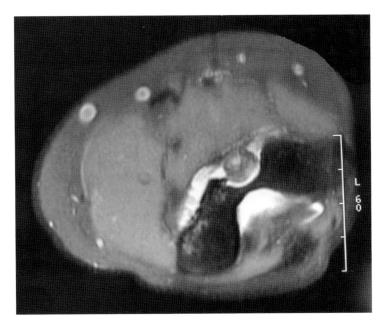

Figure 33 An axial MRI or CT can help to clarify the location of the loose body, especially if the majority of it is not ossified, but cartilaginous

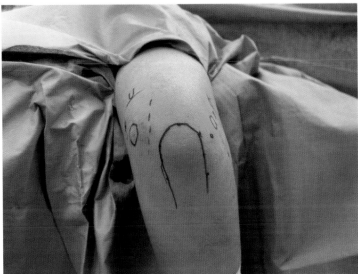

Figure 34 The position of the elbow for elbow arthroscopy. The patient may either be placed prone (as shown here) with the arm draped over a bolster on the table, or supine with the arm suspended with a holding device. The landmarks are identified and marked to avoid injury to the numerous neurovascular structures that lie within close proximity to the portal sites

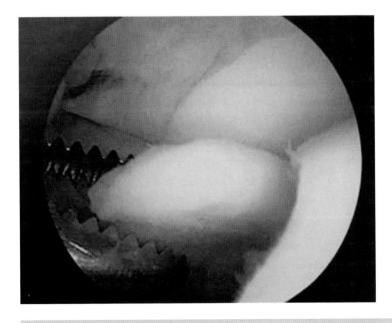

Figure 35 Arthroscopic photograph of the removal of a loose body. A grasper with teeth is inserted and used to secure the loose body. The grasper is then gently twisted out through the portal. Often, the portal needs to be enlarged to extract the loose body in its entirety

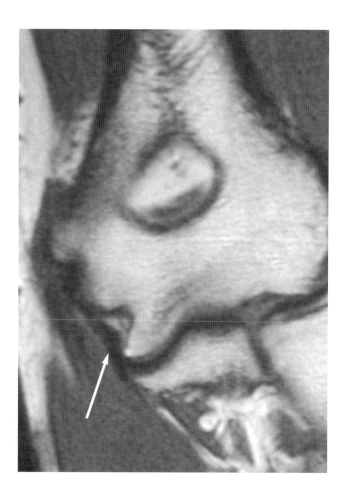

Figure 36 A coronal oblique MRI of a patient's elbow, illustrating a normal medial collateral ligament. The ligament runs from the medial epicondyle to the sublime tubercle of the ulna and provides stability to the elbow under conditions of valgus stress (such as in the pitching motion)

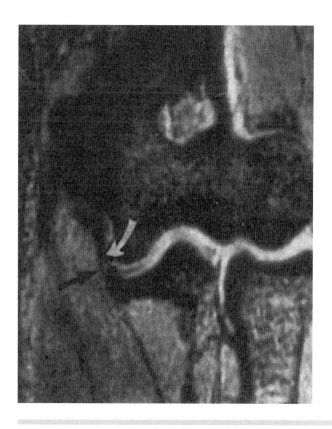

Figure 37 This is also a coronal oblique MRI (T2-weighted) that shows a disruption of the medial collateral ligament as it courses from the humerus to the ulna. Depending on the MRI protocol used, an MRI arthrogram may provide more information about the competency of the ligament

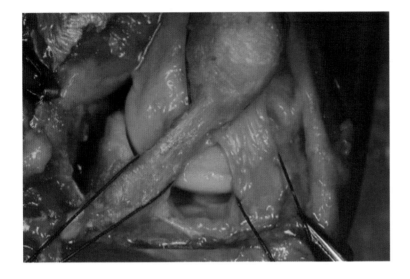

Figure 38 An anatomic dissection of a cadaver elbow showing the anterior and posterior bundles of the medial collateral ligament and their respective attachment sites. In extension, the anterior bundle becomes taut and, in flexion, the posterior bundle becomes taut, thus providing stability to the elbow throughout its range of motion

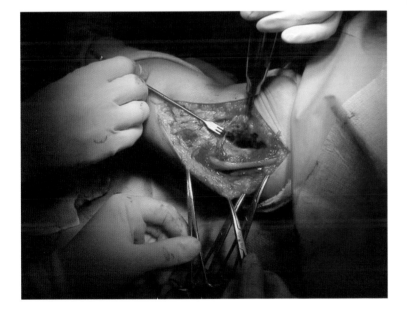

Figure 39 This intraoperative photograph demonstrates the close proximity of the ulnar nerve to the medial collateral ligament and the need to identify the nerve so as to protect it throughout the operation when reconstructing the medial collateral ligament.

Pitchers and other athletes in throwing sports place a great deal of stress across the medial collateral ligament. Athletes with injuries to the medial collateral ligament will generally complain of medial elbow pain and a decrease in their ability to throw hard. The more common differential diagnoses for patients with medial elbow pain include: medial collateral ligament insufficiency, ulnar nerve compression, flexor–pronator tendonitis (golfer's elbow) and posteromedial overload syndrome. The medial collateral ligament symptoms can often be reproduced with a valgus stress test called the milking maneuver. Ulnar nerve dysfunction usually radiates distally to the 4th and 5th fingers and can be seen concomitantly with medial collateral ligament dysfunction. In these cases, the ulnar nerve is often transposed at the time of the medial collateral ligament reconstruction

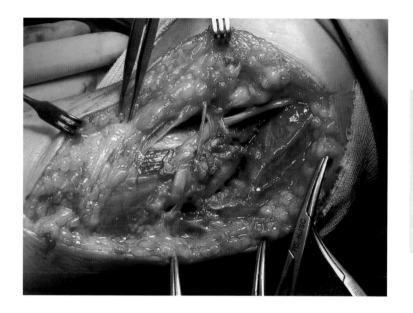

Figure 40 Intraoperative photograph of a subcutaneous ulnar nerve transposition. This can be performed for isolated ulnar nerve compression or in concert with an medial collateral ligament reconstruction in athletes who are having symptoms of ulnar neuritis in addition to their medial collateral ligament insufficiency

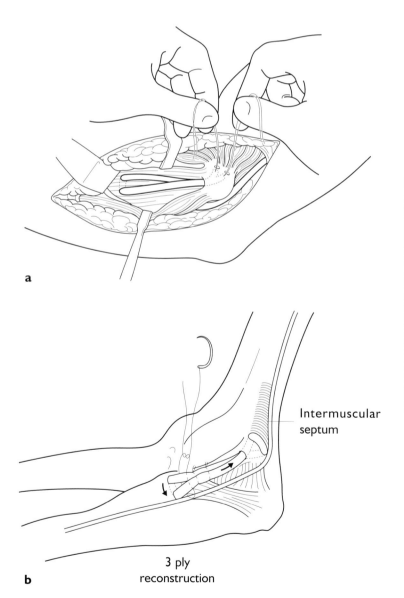

a

Intermuscular
septum

b   3 ply
    reconstruction

Figures 41 These diagrams illustrate two different techniques used to reconstruct the medial collateral ligament. (a) The technique popularized by Dr Frank Jobe was the initial procedure performed on patients with medial collateral ligament pathology; (b) the docking procedure, a modification of the same operation, was popularized by Dr David Altchek. Both procedures use an autograft palmaris tendon to reconstruct, through a series of drill holes, the medial collateral ligament and to restore valgus stability to the elbow

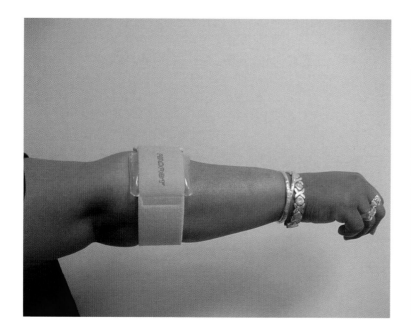

Figure 42 Clinical photograph of a patient with lateral epicondylitis (tendonitis of the extensor carpi radialis brevis). Commonly called tennis elbow, this degenerative condition is more appropriately described by the term tendinosis. Microtearing of the extensor carpi radialis brevis and granulation tissue perpetuate the cycle of repeated injury to the origin of this tendon. Activity modification, oral anti-inflammatory medicines, stretching exercises, physical therapy, and braces, such as the one pictured, can help to speed the recovery time. The band pictured here is intended to blunt the force of the muscle before it reaches the lateral epicondyle where the tendon originates

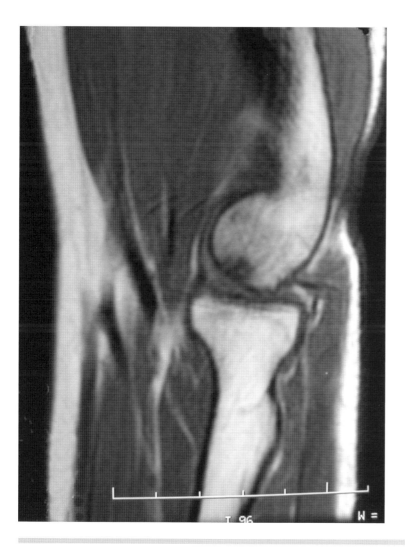

Figure 43 Sagittal MRI of a patient with an osteochondritis dessicans lesion (OCD) of the capitellum. These lesions usually involve separation of the overlying cartilage from the subchondral bone. The bone does not light up like the rest of the bone, indicating a problem with its blood supply and viability. The most common place for this lesion in the elbow is the capitellum. This patient's symptoms included pain and locking of the elbow with throwing. The lesion is often seen in children with open growth plates, and these patients have the best prognosis. They are treated with activity modification and anti-inflammatory medicines. If a loose fragment is seen, then surgical intervention is recommended to either fix the fragment back into place or to excise the loose body and stimulate the underlying bone to achieve fibrocartilagenous ingrowth

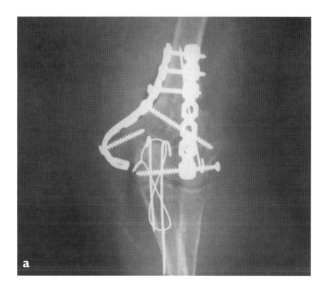

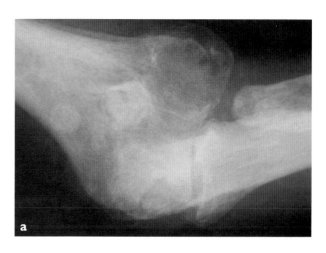

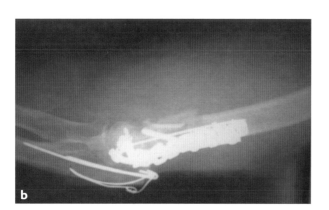

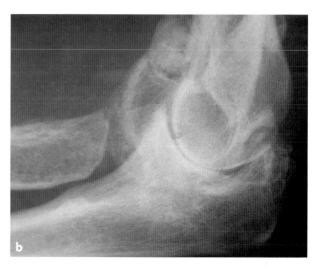

Figure 44   Anteroposterior (a) and lateral (b) radiographs of an adult patient who sustained a comminuted supracondylar fracture. The patient underwent open reduction and internal fixation for this fracture with both medial and posterolateral column plating to create the most stable construct and allow for an early range of motion. The most common complication after an elbow fracture is stiffness and so the fixation of any elbow fracture should be strong enough to allow early motion

Figure 45   Anteroposterior (a) and lateral (b) radiographs showing a patient who developed post-traumatic degenerative joint disease after an intra-articular fracture. These patients have a very limited and painful range of motion and it can often affect their ability to perform activities of daily living

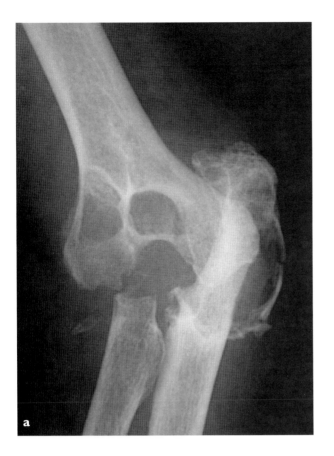

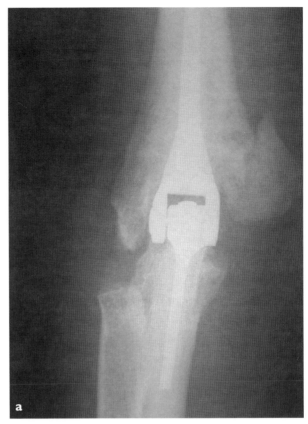

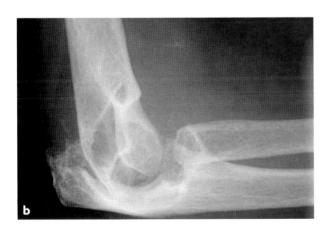

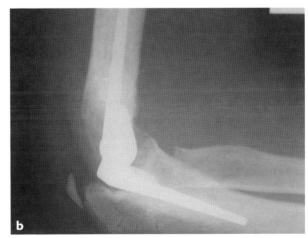

Figure 46 Anteroposterior (a) and lateral (b) radiographs of a patient with rheumatoid arthritis causing degenerative joint disease of her elbow. Rheumatoid patients often end up with multiple joint replacements due to the early and aggressive nature of their disease

Figure 47 Anteroposterior (a) and lateral (b) radiographs of a patient who underwent a total elbow arthroplasty. The treatment for degenerative disease of the elbow (whether post-traumatic arthritis, osteoarthritis, or rheumatoid arthritis) is debridement versus a total elbow arthroplasty. Debridements and releases will often improve motion, but the motion may be associated with increased pain due to the lack of underlying cartilage. Total elbow arthroplasties are becoming more popular as technology improves

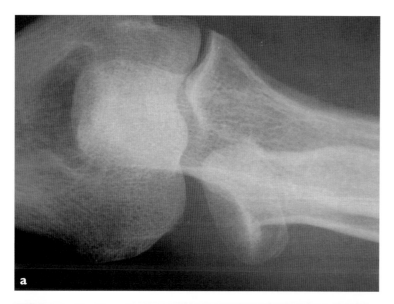

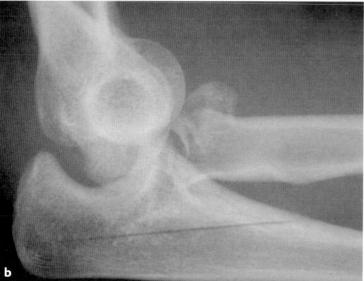

Figure 48 Anteroposterior (a) and lateral (b) radiographs of a patient who sustained a traumatic displaced radial neck fracture. These fractures can be associated with injury to the posterior interosseous nerve (PIN) due to its proximity to the radial neck. For the same reasons, if surgical intervention is chosen, care must be taken to protect the PIN from injury

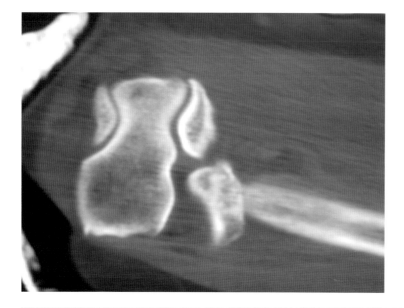

Figure 49 CT scan illustrating the radial neck fracture and better visualizing the articular surface for careful pre-operative planning

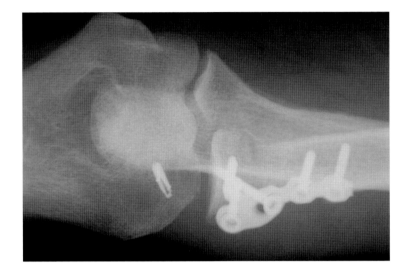

Figure 50 Anteroposterior postoperative radiograph showing the reduction and internal fixation of the radial neck fracture and a suture anchor proximally in the lateral epicondyle to repair the lateral collateral ligament

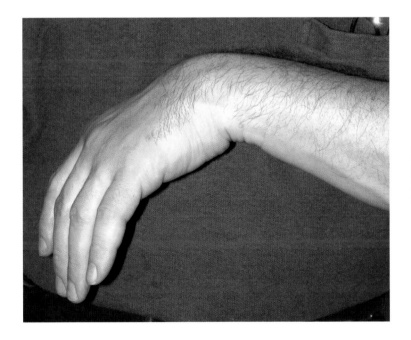

Figure 51 Clinical picture of a patient with a PIN palsy

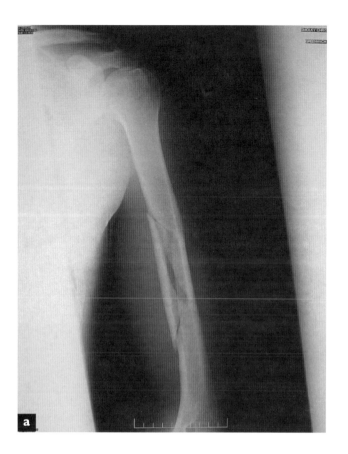

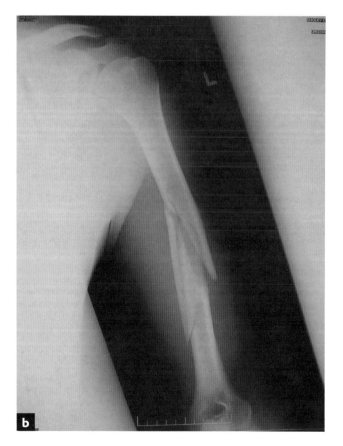

Figure 52 Anteroposterior (a) and oblique (b) radiographs of a patient with a comminuted humeral shaft fracture. The patient sustained this spiral fracture while pitching in a baseball game. Humeral shaft fractures generally heal well with non-operative management. Treatment with a Sarmiento-type brace usually yields adequate alignment and healing. Operative indications for humeral shaft fractures include: patients with polytrauma, open fractures, vascular injuries, closed-head injury and pathologic fractures. Radial nerve injuries can be seen with humeral shaft fractures (less than 10%). The rate of non-union is higher with operative treatment than with non-operative treatment in these fractures. This patient went on to heal the fracture in approximately 12 weeks and was back pitching by 5 months

Chapter 3

The shoulder

ANATOMY

The shoulder is a complex joint involving the proximal humerus, the scapula and the clavicle. The glenohumeral articulation has the greatest range of motion of any joint in the body. It is not only the least constrained joint, but, as a result, it is also the most unstable joint in the body, with the most reported dislocations.

The greater and lesser tuberosities of the proximal humerus serve as attachment sites for the rotator cuff tendons. It is the deforming forces of these tendons that may be responsible for tuberosity displacement in proximal humerus fractures. The acromioclavicular joint is very superficial and thus susceptible to injury by direct impact. The acromioclavicular joint often remains subluxed or even dislocated after injury.

The main stability to the glenohumeral joint is afforded by the capsulo-ligamentous structures and the rotator cuff muscles. The capsule and ligaments play an important role in the static stability of the shoulder. It is this complex that is often injured when the shoulder is dislocated, the so-called Bankart lesion (avulsion of the inferior glenohumeral ligament). Dynamic stability is afforded by the rotator cuff muscles, the subscapularis, supraspinatus, infraspinatus and teres minor.

The shoulder is subject to a variety of pathologic conditions including fractures, dislocations and instability, impingement, rotator cuff disease and degenerative joint disease.

HISTORY AND PHYSICAL EXAMINATION

Shoulder pathology can present in a variety of ways. Fractures and dislocations are relatively easy to diagnose and are usually seen in the emergency room setting. Impingement, subtle instability, rotator cuff pathology and degenerative disease often develop more insidiously and therefore require a detailed history and thorough examination to make the correct diagnosis. In addition, several medical conditions and other musculoskeletal pathologies can masquerade as shoulder pain. The cervical spine can often cause radicular shoulder pain. Conditions that irritate the phrenic nerve can also lead to shoulder pain, such as myocardial infarction, subphrenic abscesses, or pneumonias.

Physical examination should start with inspection and palpation. Findings such as atrophy of the deltoid or rotator cuff or bulging of the biceps from rupture of the long head may be readily apparent on inspection. The range of motion is then checked against the normal side and manual muscle testing should be performed on all major muscles and muscle groups about the shoulder. Discrepancies between passive and active motion may be a clue to tendon rupture (rotator cuff) or neurological lesions. Painful stiffness may occur both with degenerative joint changes (arthritis) or intra-articular inflammation and scarring (frozen shoulder). Inferior instability may be demonstrated by checking for a positive sulcus sign; anterior instability can be checked by abducting the arm and externally rotating it to elicit apprehension from the patient.

DIAGNOSTIC STUDIES

Plain radiographs are very useful in diagnosing shoulder pathology. Anteroposterior, axillary and outlet views should be obtained in all cases of trauma. The axillary view enables the clinician to diagnose an anterior or posterior dislocation which can otherwise be overlooked. Lesions associated with dislocations (i.e. Bankart and Hill–Sachs) can also be seen on the axillary view. The outlet view is helpful in assessing acromial morphology which can be the cause of impingement syndromes. Calcific tendonitis can be demonstrated on the anterioposterior views (sometimes internal rotation and external rotation views can be helpful). Acromioclavicular separations and proximal humerus fractures are also diagnosed by plain radiographs. Osteoarthritis is demonstrated by diminished joint space and the presence of classic inferior osteophytes.

MRI and ultrasonography may be extremely useful in evaluation of soft tissue injuries about the shoulder. Bankart lesions can be evaluated, as well as biceps or rotator cuff pathology. Most diagnoses can be made based on a careful history, physical examination and the use of plain radiographs. MRI should be used to confirm the diagnosis if questions exist.

DISORDERS

The most common disorders about the shoulder are illustrated in Figures 53–93.

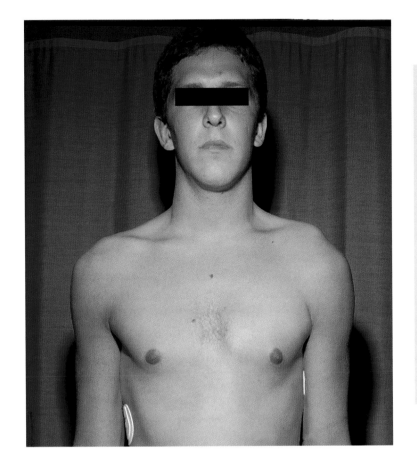

Figure 53 Clinical photograph of a young man who fell and sustained a direct impact to the right shoulder, causing an acromioclavicular (AC) separation. AC separations are divided into six types, based on the ligaments ruptured and the amount and direction of displacement. A type I injury is a non-displaced sprain of the AC ligament, a type II injury is a rupture of the AC ligament with minimal displacement, a type III injury is disruption of both the AC ligament as well as the coracoclavicular ligaments with resulting displacement between 25 and 100%, a type IV injury is a posterior dislocation, a type V injury is a type III with associated rupture of the delto-trapezial fascia and displacement of 100–300%, and a type VI injury is an inferior dislocation of the clavicle

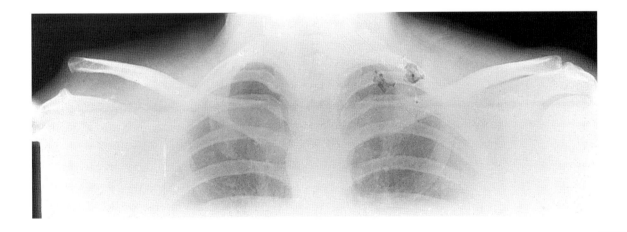

Figure 54 Anteroposterior weighted radiograph demonstrates more than 100% displacement, indicating a type V injury to the acromioclavicular joint

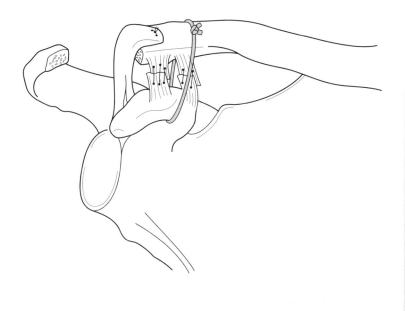

Figure 55 To avoid continued pain and decreased strength and stability, the type V separations are reconstructed in a modified Weaver–Dunn fashion. This diagram illustrates the technique used. The coracoacromial ligament is taken with as much length as possible off the acromion and transferred to the end of the clavicle. Approximately 5 mm of the distal clavicle is removed, drill holes are created and the coracoacromial ligament is tied down to the distal clavicle with the acromioclavicular joint reduced. Before the final repair is tied, a suture or piece of merciline tape is brought around the base of the coracoid and tied over the distal clavicle to take tension off the newly reconstructed ligament, in order to facilitate healing. Most often, the ruptured coracoclavicular ligaments are not visible, but, if present, should be repaired to strengthen the construct

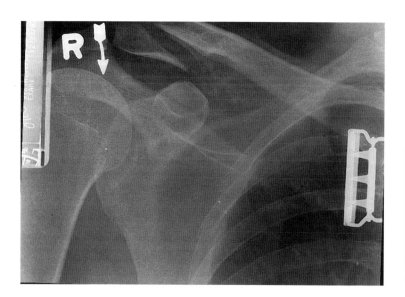

Figure 56 Anteroposterior radiograph of a distal clavicle fracture. Clavicle fractures are classified by the location of the fracture. Type I fractures are in the middle third of the shaft and constitute the majority of clavicle fractures. Type II fractures are in the distal third and are further subdivided, based on ligament disruption and resulting instability of the clavicle. The type II fractures that result in instability should be treated with open reduction with internal fixation. Type III fractures are in the medial third. Most clavicle fractures heal uneventfully, despite deformity and angulation, with sling immobilization for 6–8 weeks

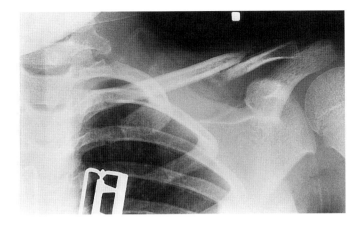

Figure 57 Anteroposterior radiograph of the right shoulder demonstrating a mid-third clavicle shaft fracture with shortening and overlap. The patient was treated with a sling and went on to heal this fracture without complication

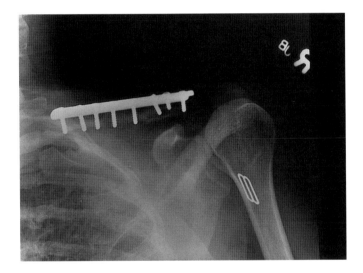

Figure 58 Anteroposterior radiograph of an open reduction with internal fixation of a clavicle performed for a painful non-union. Most clavicle fractures heal without the need for surgical intervention. However, there are a few indications for open reduction and internal fixation. Acutely, open fractures, fractures that cause skin tenting, and fractures associated with vascular injury are treated with open reduction with internal fixation. The rates of non-union for all clavicle fractures are low. Symptomatic non-unions are treated with open reduction with internal fixation

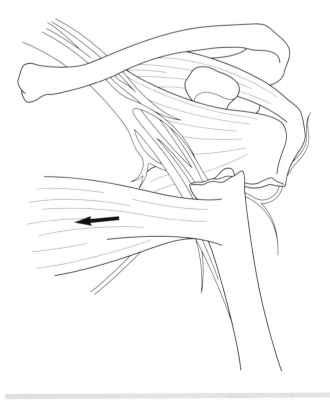

Figure 59 Diagram representing the major musculotendinous deforming forces on proximal humerus fractures

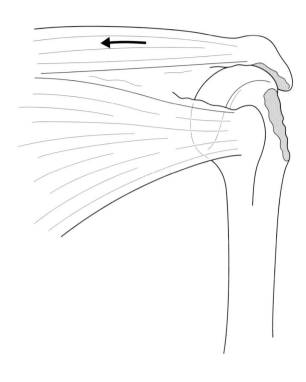

Figure 60   Diagram of a greater tuberosity fracture with the supraspinatus pulling the fracture posteriorly and superiorly

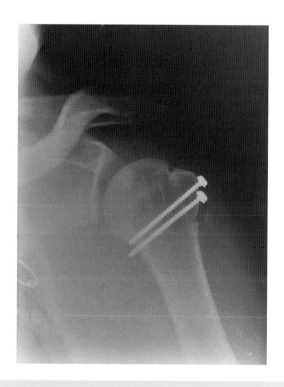

Figure 62   Anteroposterior radiograph of a greater tuberosity fracture treated with open reduction with internal fixation. The indications for open reduction with internal fixation of greater tuberosity fractures are narrower than those for other proximal humerus fractures due to the impingement that can occur with minimal displacement. Open reduction with internal fixation should be considered if the displacement is greater than 5 mm

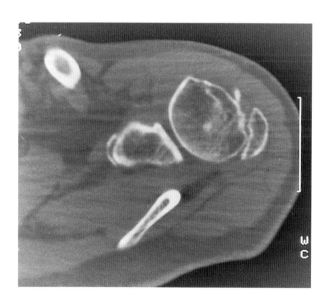

Figure 61   Axial CT scan of a patient illustrating posterior displacement of the greater tuberosity

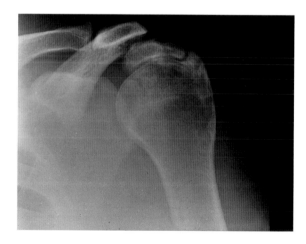

Figure 63   Anteroposterior radiograph of a patient who sustained a greater tuberosity fracture. The patient did not receive operative treatment and the fracture subsequently healed in a superiorly displaced position, causing the patient significant pain and limitation with abduction and forward flexion

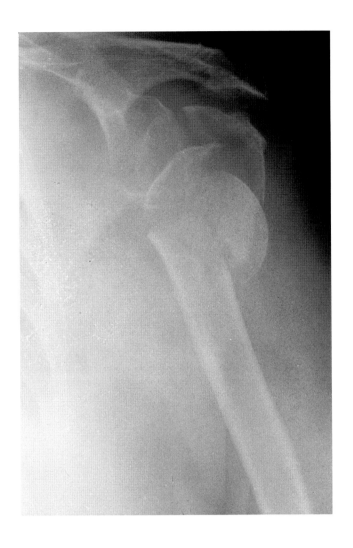

Figure 64 Anteroposterior radiograph of a four-part proximal humeral fracture. The four parts are the humeral shaft, the greater tuberosity, the lesser tuberosity and the humeral head. Neer defined a part as any fracture fragment with more than 1-cm displacement or 45° of angulation. Four-part fractures place the humeral head at extremely high risk for avascular necrosis since it jeapordizes the major blood supply, the anterior humeral circumflex artery. Because of the high risk of avascular necrosis, most four-part fractures are treated with hemi-arthroplasty

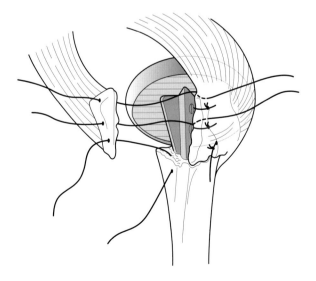

Figure 65 Diagram illustrating the technique for hemi-arthroplasty in four-part proximal humeral fractures. The tuberosities are attached to the prosthesis, each other and the shaft with strong, non-absorbable suture. Bone grafting of the tuberosities from the humeral head can help the tuberosities heal to the shaft (non-union of the tuberosities is the major complication following this operation)

AN ATLAS OF ORTHOPEDIC SURGERY

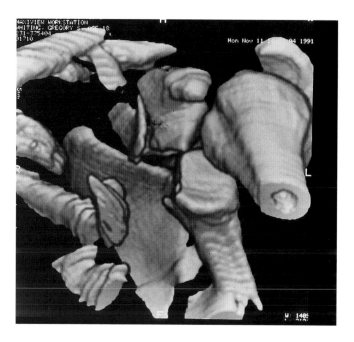

Figure 66 Three-dimensional CT scan of a comminuted scapula/glenoid fracture. These injuries are usually high-energy injuries and other concomitant injuries should be suspected (e.g. lung injuries and vascular injuries). Three-dimensional CT scans can be very useful in these complex fractures to determine the number of parts and displacement prior to deciding on a treatment plan

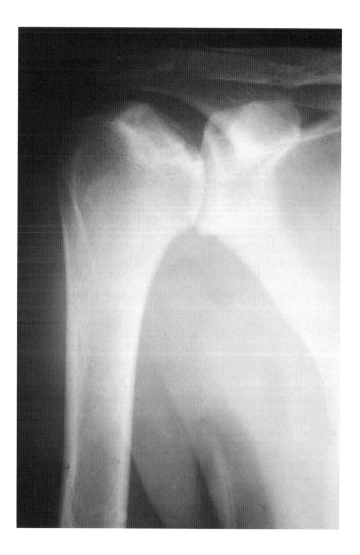

Figure 67 Anteroposterior radiograph of a patient with significant shoulder pain. The radiograph demonstrates collapse and deformity of the humeral head associated with advanced avascular necrosis. Avascular necrosis is associated with steroid use, alcoholism, and sickle-cell anemia. Treatment for avascular necrosis of the humeral head depends on the stage and glenoid involvement. If there is humeral head collapse and glenoid involvement, a total shoulder arthroplasty will provide the best pain relief for the patient

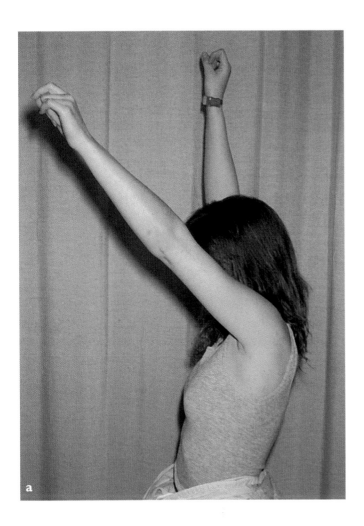

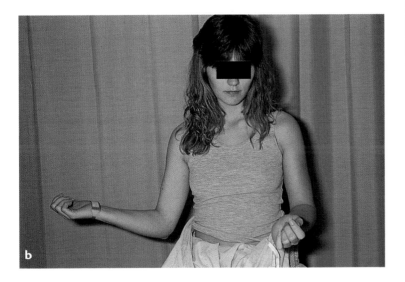

Figure 68   Clinical photographs of a young patient with a severely limited range of motion in both forward flexion (a) and external rotation (b). In young patients with limited motion, the clinician must differentiate restriction of motion secondary to pain, seen in patients with impingement, versus true mechanical restriction to motion from the scarred capsule, seen in patients with adhesive capsulitis (frozen shoulder). In patients with restriction in external rotation, a high suspicion of frozen shoulder should be maintained. Patients with impingement rarely have restriction to external rotation and more commonly are limited in internal rotation. A diagnostic sub-acromial injection of lidocaine will relieve the pain associated with impingement and should allow normal range of motion. If the patient continues to have restricted motion despite the injection, then a frozen shoulder should be considered in the differential diagnosis

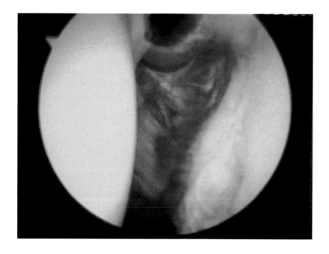

Figure 69 Patients with adhesive capsulitis who do not respond to gleno-humeral steroid injections followed by physical therapy may need to undergo manipulation under anesthesia and arthroscopic capsular release in order to regain their motion. This arthroscopic picture demonstrates the severe capsuli-tis that is present in patients with painful frozen shoulders

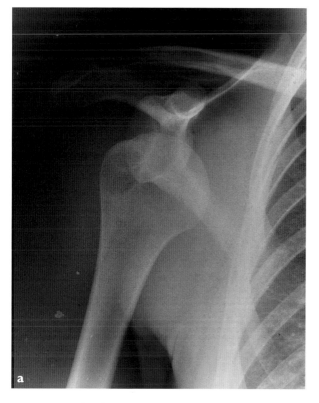

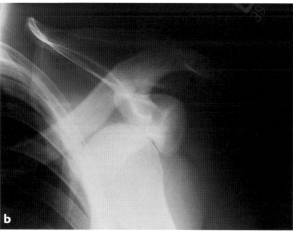

Figure 70 Anteroposterior (a) and outlet (b) radiographs demonstrating an acute anterior shoulder dislocation. The glenohumeral joint is the most commonly dislocated joint in the body. The restrictions to dislocation are the bony articulation, the labrum, the capsule and the rotator cuff. The likeli-hood of re-dislocation is based on the patient's age at first dislocation. Patients under 20 years old have better than a 90% chance of re-dislocation. Acute traumatic dislocations usually result in an injury to the inferior glenohumeral ligament, the so-called Bankart lesion. Patients with traumatic dislocations and Bankart lesions do well with surgical repair of the labrum to the glenoid

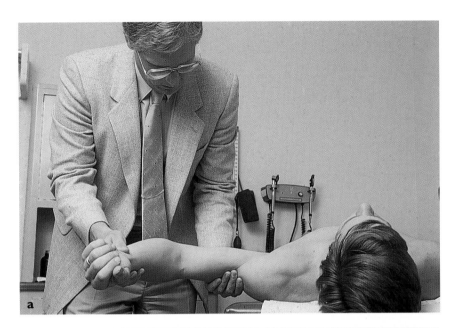

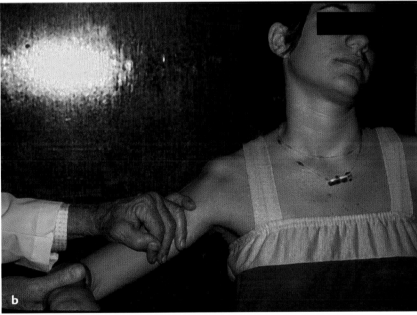

Figure 71   Provocative maneuvers are performed on patients with a history of instability. The apprehension test (a) places the arm in 90° of abduction and 90° of external rotation. A positive test is seen in patients who complain that their shoulder feels as if it might dislocate. The inferior sulcus sign (b) is seen in patients with generalized ligamentous laxity. It is important to differentiate patients with traumatic dislocations from those patients with generalized ligamentous laxity and underlying multidirectional instability (MDI). Patients with MDI should be treated with rehabilitation of the rotator cuff and scapulo-thoracic strengthening. Surgery is a last resort in these patients, and, when indicated, should address the capsular laxity that is the underlying pathology

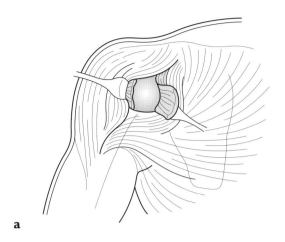
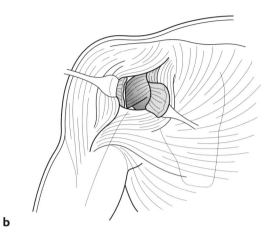

a   b

Figures 72   Diagrams of an anterior capsular shift. The capsule is separated from the subscapularis muscle (a) and then divided in a horizontal fashion. The inferior flap is shifted superior-laterally and the superior flap is shifted infero-laterally (b), removing the redundancy in the capsular tissue

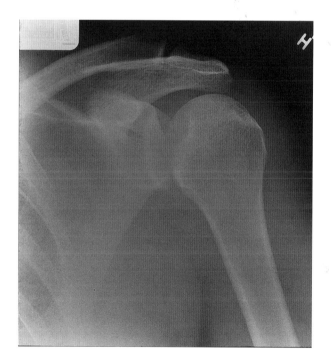

Figure 73   Anteroposterior radiograph of a patient who sustained an injury to his right shoulder. This radiograph can be deceptive in cases of posterior dislocations. An axillary radiograph or axial CT is necessary to confirm the diagnosis

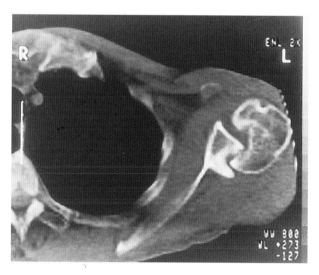

Figure 74   Axial CT of the same patient demonstrating a posterior locked humeral dislocation. These dislocations can be reduced under anesthesia. If the shoulder cannot be reduced closed, then an open reduction is performed

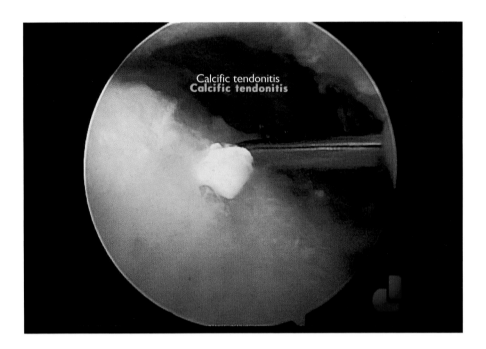

Figure 75   Arthroscopic picture of calcium deposits in the supraspinatus tendon. Calcific tendonitis is an extremely painful condition that has the appearance of impingement on physical examination. Radiographs will sometimes show the calcium deposits in the tendon. Calcific tendonitis will usually respond to aspiration of the calcium, injection of steroids and rehabilitation exercises for the rotator cuff. If non-operative management fails, then arthroscopic debridement and acromioplasty are indicated

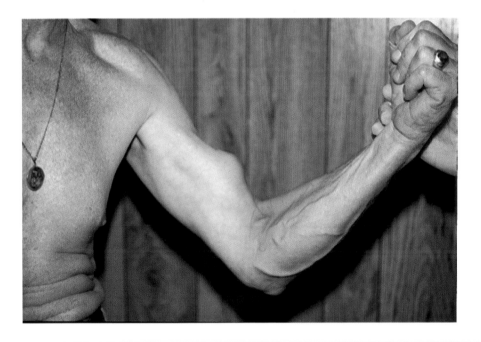

Figure 76   Clinical photograph of a patient with a rupture to the proximal biceps. The rupture was preceded by several months of pain in the bicipital groove. Rupture of the biceps relieved his pain and left him with the cosmetic deformity shown (the popeye lesion). There is minimal loss of strength (approximately 10%) in both flexion and supination; however, patients may complain of cramping pain in the muscle belly

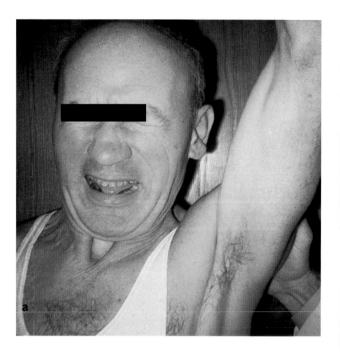

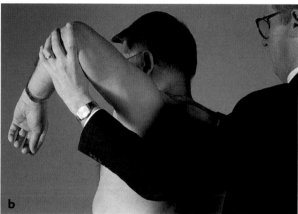

Figure 77   Clinical photographs illustrating the Neer (a) and Hawkins (b) tests for impingement. These tests are provocative maneuvers causing the supraspinatus tendon to impinge under the acromion and further aggravate the bursal inflammation and pain

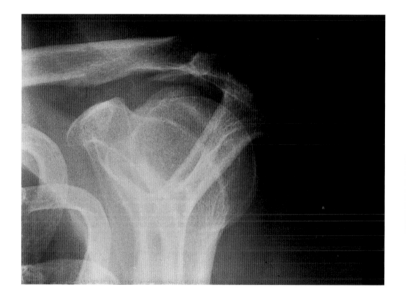

Figure 78   Outlet view of the shoulder demonstrating the anterolateral acromial spur that is often seen in patients with impingement. Acromial morphology is divided into three types. Type I is a flat acromion, type II is a curved acromion, and type III is a hooked acromion. This radiograph shows the most common type II acromion

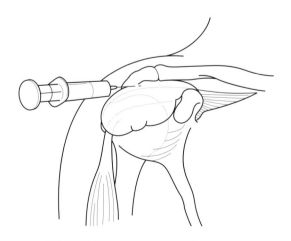

Figure 79   Illustration of a diagnostic subacromial injection into the bursa. Cortisone can also be added to the injection to make it both diagnostic and therapeutic

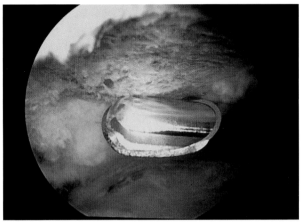

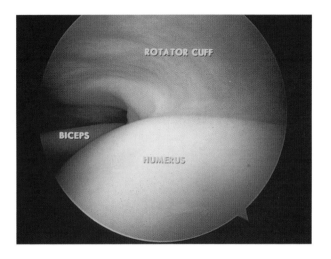

Figure 80 Patients with impingement who do not respond to physical therapy (rotator cuff strengthening) and cortisone injections may elect to undergo arthroscopic subacromial decompression. This arthroscopic photograph shows the undersurface of the acromion after removal of the spur with a full-radius shaver

Figure 81 Arthroscopic photograph of a normal rotator cuff attachment on the articular side

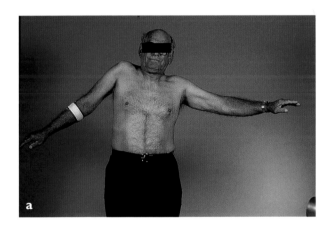

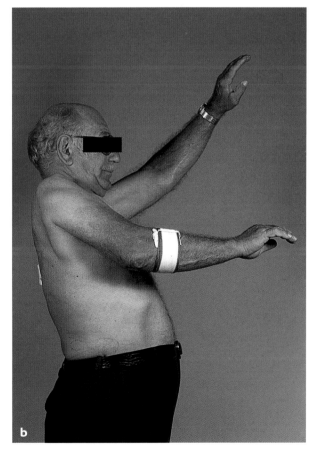

Figure 82 Clinical photographs of a patient with a massive rotator cuff tear. The patient has a positive 'shrug' sign, in both abduction (a) and forward flexion (b). He uses scapulo-thoracic motion to compensate for his inability to elevate the arm through the glenohumeral joint

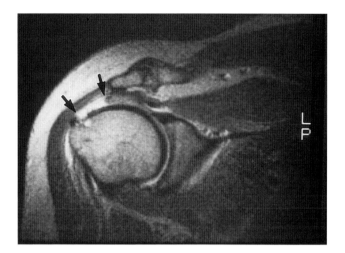

Figure 83   Coronal oblique MRI of a supraspinatus tear with retraction

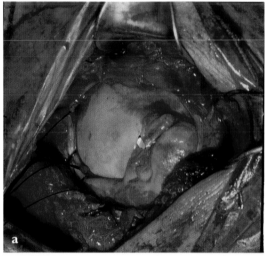

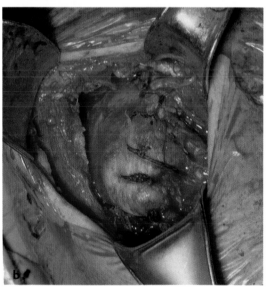

Figure 84   Intraoperative photographs of a massive rotator cuff tear with exposed humeral head (a), and after repair with complete coverage and approximation of the tendon back to the greater tuberosity (b)

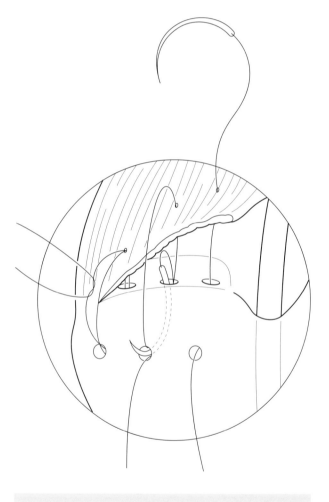

Figure 85   Diagram illustrating the technique for rotator cuff repair using drill holes through the tuberosity. With newer technology, many surgeons now choose suture anchors, even when performing open rotator cuff repairs

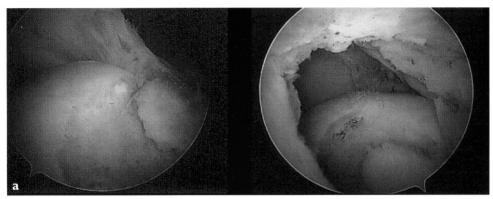

Intra-articular   Bursal view

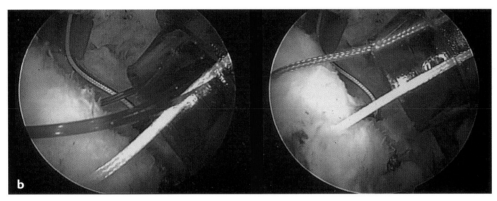

Place second suture anchor and pass suture through cuff

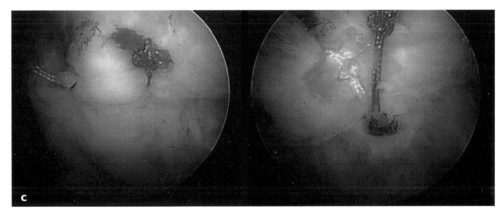

Repeat with additional anchors, from back to front, to achieve final repair

Figure 86   Arthroscopic identification of a rotator cuff tear. The ends of the cuff are debrided and freshened and the bony bed is prepared by decortication. The decision on whether to repair the rotator cuff arthroscopically or through a mini-opening is mainly based on arthroscopic skills. Larger cuff tears which used to be repaired with an open operation are more amenable to arthroscopic repair thanks to newer instrument designs that have made suture placement much easier

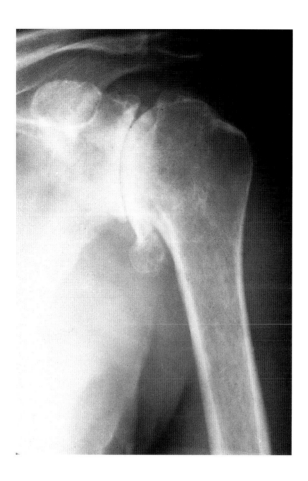

Figure 87 Anteroposterior radiograph of a patient with advanced degenerative disease of the glenohumeral joint. The classic inferior humeral osteophyte is present at the base of the humeral head, and the joint space is obliterated with subchondral sclerosis present on both the humeral head and glenoid. Often, it is useful to have a good axillary radiograph or axial CT to determine the wear pattern on the glenoid for preoperative planning

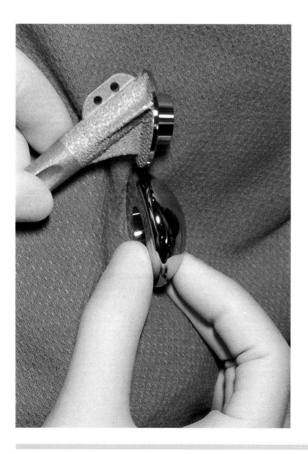

Figure 88 A modular humeral prosthesis

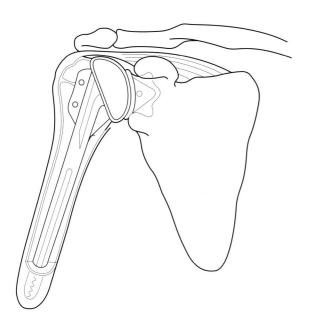

Figure 89 Diagram of a total shoulder prosthesis illustrating the relationships of the prosthesis to the bones and muscles that surround it

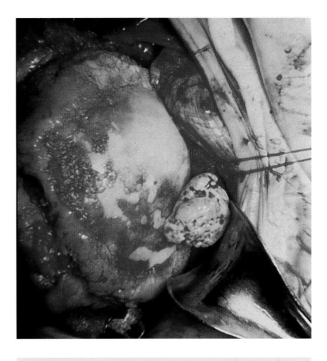

Figure 90 Intraoperative photograph of the humeral head with abundant osteophytes and loose bodies. In order to make an appropriate humeral cut, it is important to define the true humeral head by removing the osteophytes

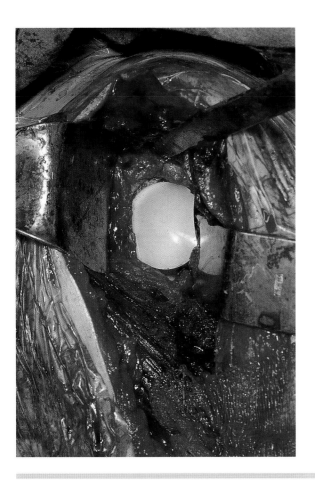

Figure 91 Intraoperative photograph of the glenoid prosthesis. This polyethylene implant is cemented into the glenoid with minimal removal of bone and should seat well against the native glenoid, with minimal motion to avoid component loosening

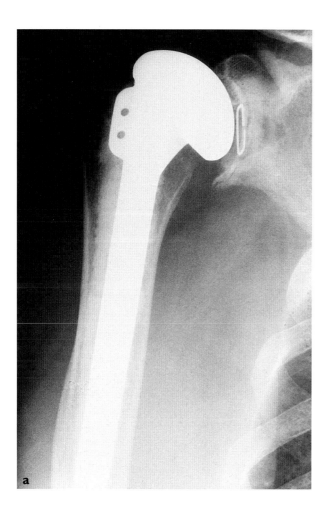

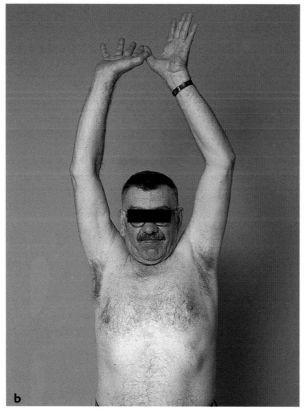

Figure 92 Anteroposterior radiograph (a) and clinical photograph (b) of a patient with a total shoulder arthroplasty for osteoarthritis. Total shoulder arthroplasty is a reliable operation for pain relief. Functional outcomes vary and depend primarily on the patient's preoperative function

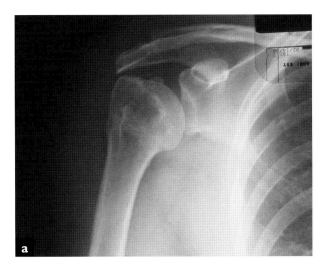

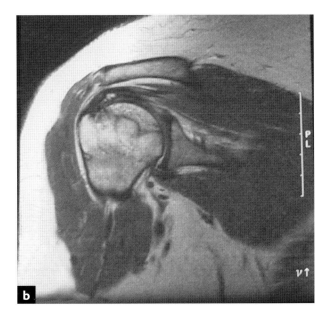

Figures 93 Anteroposterior radiograph (a) of the right shoulder demonstrating humeral head deformity and collapse. Sagittal T1 (b) and T2 (c) weighted images clearly show the advanced avascular necrosis with collapse. Patients can develop avascular necrosis from steroids, alcoholism, and sickle-cell disease. Post-traumatic avascular necrosis of the humeral head is usually associated with three- or four-part fractures in which the blood supply has been jeopardized. Treatment for avascular necrosis depends on glenoid involvement. If the glenoid is spared, a hemi-arthroplasty is often adequate. If the glenoid is involved, a total shoulder arthroplasty will offer the best pain relief

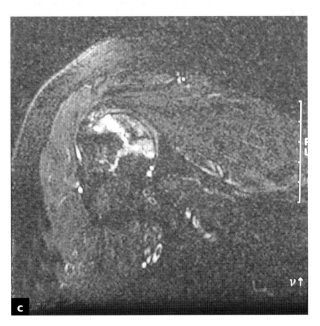

Chapter 4

The hip

ANATOMY

The hip is the most proximal joint in the lower extremity. It is a ball-and-socket joint. The femoral head (the ball) articulates with the acetabulum (the socket) in a very conforming fashion. The acetabulum is formed by the ilium, ischium and pubic bones of the pelvis. The presence of the femoral head is a necessary component to the formation of a normal acetabulum; for example, a patient with developmental dysplasia of the hip has a dysplastic acetabulum resulting from the absence of the femoral head in the socket during development. The acetabulum is deepened by the presence of a fibro-cartilagenous labrum. The hip articulation is surrounded by the joint capsule and the iliofemoral and pubofemoral ligaments anteriorly and the ischiofemoral ligament posteriorly. The ligamentum teres runs from the acetabulum into the femoral head and carries a branch of the obturator artery, which is responsible for a significant part of the vascular supply to the femoral head during development. In adults, the major blood supply to the femoral head comes from the medial circumflex artery, a branch of the femoral artery. The greater and lesser trochanters of the femur serve as attachment sites for the major muscles and tendons about the hip. The abductors insert onto the greater trochanter and the iliopsoas, a major hip flexor, onto the lesser trochanter.

HISTORY AND PHYSICAL EXAMINATION

Determination of the nature of hip pain is important. Is the pain acute, or did it develop over time?

These are important historical questions to elicit. Acute pain following a trauma can indicate a fracture, muscle strain or contusion. Insidious pain that has developed over time may lead the clinician more toward the diagnosis of enthesopathies, arthopathies, or neoplastic disorders. Where is the pain located? Groin pain usually indicates intra-articular pathology, whereas lateral-sided hip pain is more commonly associated with the enthesopathies or a trochanteric bursitis. Thigh pain and even knee pain may be referred from the hip joint.

Physical examination begins with observation of gait pattern. Trendelenberg gait may denote hip abductor weakness, while an antalgic gait may reflect degenerative hip pain. With the patient seated, motor strength can be assessed and a neurological examination can be performed. The range of motion is measured with the patient supine. The examiner must flex the contralateral hip in order to remove the lumbosacral lordosis before testing for hip extension (the Thomas maneuver). Rotation should also be carefully recorded and, as always compared to the contralateral limb. The pelvis must be stabilized with the examiner's other hand during a hip examination.

DIAGNOSTIC STUDIES

The general hip assessment should start with plain radiographs. An anteroposterior radiograph of the pelvis allows visualization of the painful hip as well as the lower lumbosacral spine, the sacroiliac joints and, most importantly, the contralateral hip.

Ultrasound is an imaging modality that is becoming more widely used in the pediatric population for assessing patients with developmental dysplasia of the hip; however, its usefulness in adults is somewhat limited. Bone scans are valuable in the diagnosis of occult hip fractures, infection and neoplasias. CT scans are very helpful in cases of pelvic trauma and the newer three-dimensional reconstructions can be invaluable in the preoperative planning for complex pelvic and acetabular fractures. MRI has the broadest capabilities. Occult hip fractures, infection, tumors, avascular necrosis, arthritis, labral tears, muscle ruptures and other soft-tissue injuries are all readily seen on MRI with increasing accuracy.

DISORDERS

The most common hip disorders are illustrated in Figures 94–112.

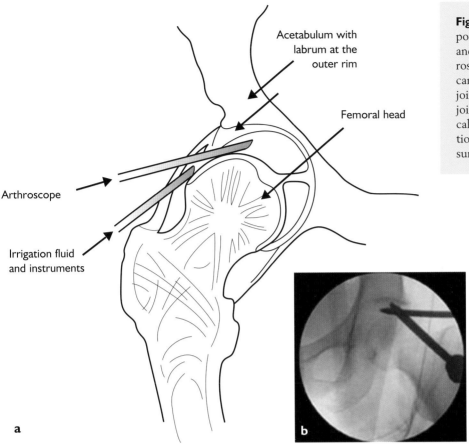

Acetabulum with
labrum at the
outer rim

Femoral head

Arthroscope

Irrigation fluid
and instruments

a

Figure 94   Diagram (a) of portals for hip arthroscopy and (b) intraoperative fluoroscopy confirming proper cannula placement in the hip joint. The hip is a difficult joint to approach arthroscopically because of its deep location in the muscles that surround it

b

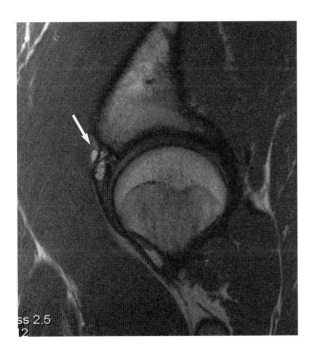

ss 2.5
2

Figure 95   Sagittal oblique MRI of a patient with pain and popping in the hip. The MRI demonstrates an anterior labral tear with cyst formation

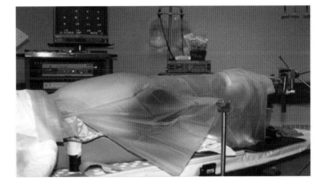

Figure 96   Lateral decubitus set-up for a hip arthroscopy. The other possible position is the supine position. The decision to use one or the other is usually based on surgeon preference. With either method, the patient is placed on the traction table with a cushioned bolster in the groin and a boot on the ipsilateral leg to allow traction to be placed across the operative hip during the procedure. Care must be taken with the amount and duration of traction, as injury to the pudendal nerve can be caused if too much traction and pressure are placed. The first portal is usually placed with arthrographic confirmation on fluoroscopy, and the subsequent portals are placed using direct arthroscopic visualization

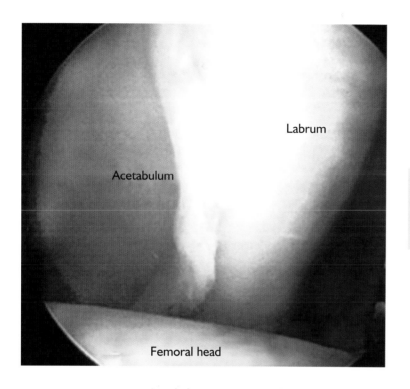

Labrum

Acetabulum

Femoral head

Figure 97 Arthroscopic photograph demonstrating the relationship of the labrum to the acetabulum and femoral head

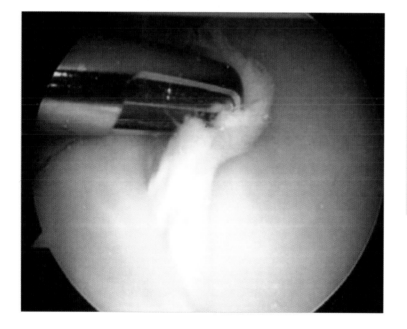

Figure 98 Arthroscopic photograph illustrating a debridement of a hip labral tear. The instrument used is an oscillating shaver. The indications for hip arthroscopy are fewer than for other joints. Indications include labral tear, loose body, synovial chondromatosis, synovial biopsies or synovectomies

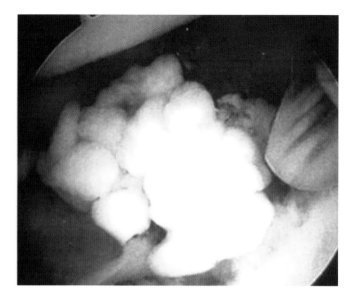

Figure 99 Arthroscopic photograph of synovial chondromatosis. Removal of the chondromatosis or other loose bodies is one of the more common indications for hip arthroscopy

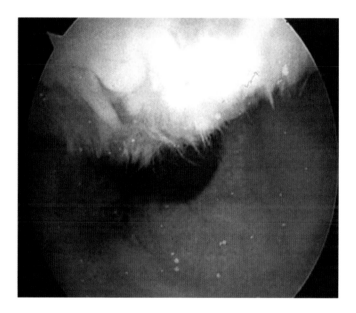

Figure 100 Arthroscopic photograph of a poor indication for hip arthroscopy. The femoral head cartilage shows advanced degeneration with fraying and fissuring, and advanced hip arthritis does not respond well to arthroscopic debridement

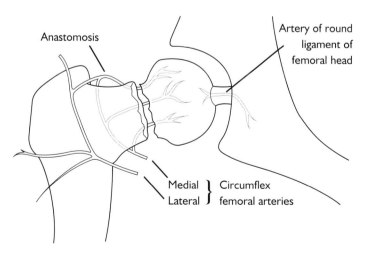

Figure 101 Knowledge of the blood supply to the femoral head is critical in deciding how to treat the different kinds of hip fractures. If the blood supply is interrupted as is the case with intracapsular fractures (e.g. displaced femoral neck fracture), the risk of avascular necrosis is high and the treatment should be aimed at replacing the femoral head with a hemi-arthroplasty. However, if the fracture is minimally displaced, or the patient is young, the surgeon may elect to fix the fracture with several screws in order to allow the fracture to heal and to preserve the patient's own femoral head

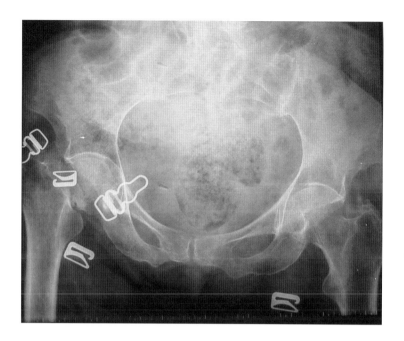

Figure 102 An example of a displaced femoral neck fracture in an elderly woman. The right hip is somewhat obscured by the clips, but one can still clearly see that the femoral neck is fractured and that the femoral head has remained seated in the acetabulum, while the femoral shaft has migrated proximally, causing the appearance of a shortened and externally rotated leg when the patient is seen in the emergency room setting

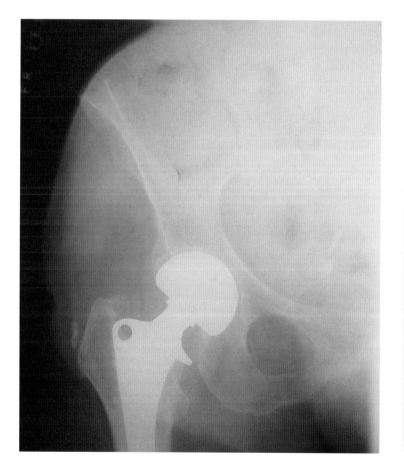

Figure 103 Postoperative radiograph of the same patient. A hemi-arthroplasty was elected in this patient to minimize the risk of a second operation (as would be the case if the fracture was fixed and the femoral head developed avascular necrosis) and to allow for immediate postoperative weight bearing.

In elderly patients with hip fractures, it is vital that the patients are out of bed and walking as soon as possible to minimize the risk of complications. The more common and serious complications associated with hip fractures include pneumonia, deep venous thrombosis and pulmonary embolus. Early mobilization and good respiratory therapy can help to minimize the risk of pneumonia. Anticoagulation is an important part of minimizing the risk of deep venous thrombosis and subsequent pulmonary embolus. Thromboembolic prophylaxis with agents such as Fragmin is common in the peri-operative period, when the risk of clot formation is highest

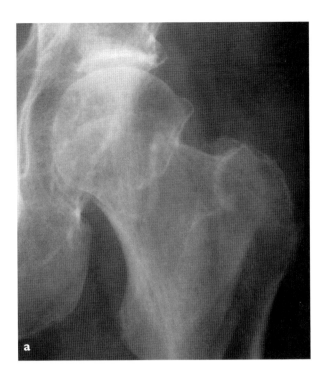
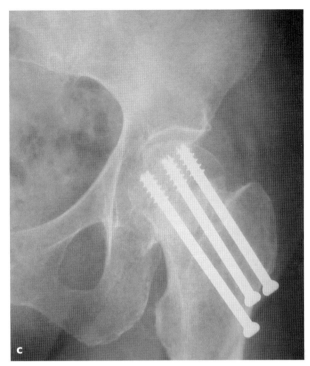
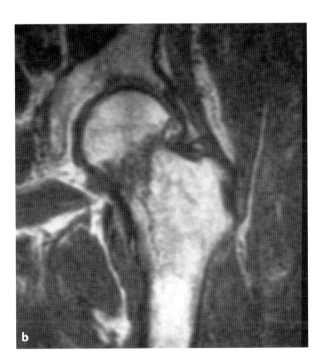
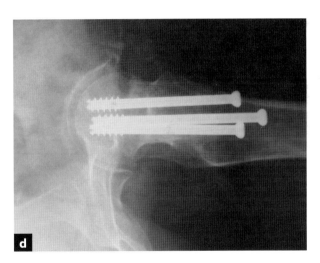

Figure 104   Pre-operative anteroposterior radiograph (a) and coronal MRI (b) demonstrate an impacted valgus femoral neck fracture. Anteroposterior (c) and lateral (d) radiographs of the same patient show treatment with a percutaneous hip pinning with three cannulated screws. This arrangement of screws gives the fracture the most stability to allow for early weight-bearing and ambulation

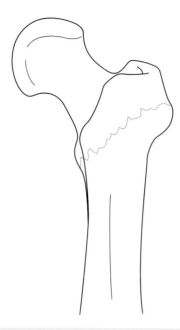

Figure 105 Diagram illustrating the anatomy and orientation of an intertrochanteric hip fracture. These are extracapsular fractures and do not disrupt the blood supply to the same degree as do the intra-capsular femoral neck fractures. These fractures are treated with a sliding hip screw and side plate to allow compression of the fracture with weight-bearing

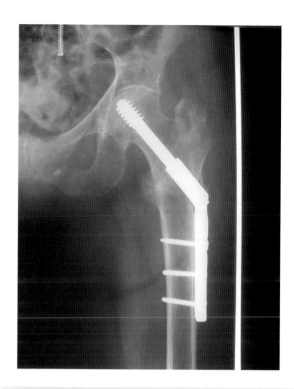

Figure 107 Postoperative radiograph of the same patient who underwent an open reduction and internal fixation with a sliding hip screw and side plate. It is important to restore the normal valgus angle of the hip prior to fixation

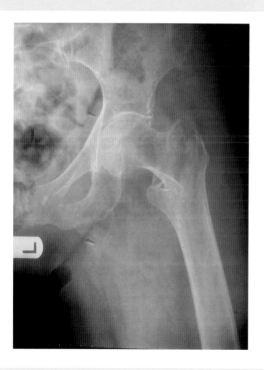

Figure 106 Anteroposterior radiograph of a patient with an intertrochanteric fracture. Note that the proximal fracture fragment goes into varus due to the muscular attachments

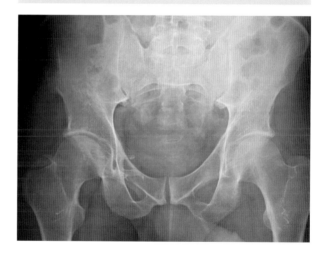

Figure 108 Anteroposterior radiograph of an elderly patient who fell at home and was unable to bear full weight on the right leg when seen in the emergency room. Though the radiograph is negative for a fracture, one should have a very high suspicion for an occult hip fracture in this setting. The patient had pain with internal rotation and heel strike and was unable to maintain a straight leg raise. The decision was made to obtain a magnetic resonance image (a bone scan can also be used) to look for an occult hip fracture

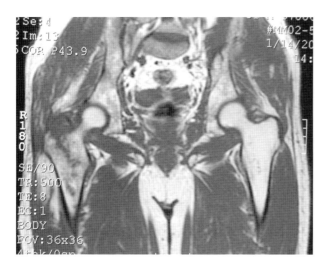

Figure 109 The MRI is positive for an intertrochanteric hip fracture of the right hip. Note the decreased signal on the TI-weighted image extending inferomedially from the greater trochanter

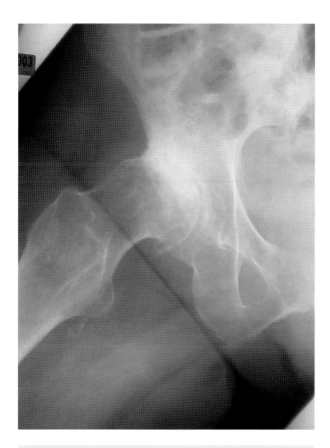

Figure 110 Anteroposterior radiograph of a patient with long-standing hip pain and limited motion. The radiograph clearly demonstrates the decreased joint space, the subchondral sclerosis and cysts indicative of advanced osteoarthritis

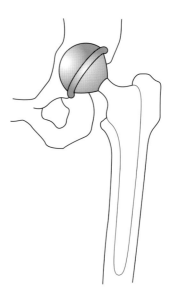

Figure 111 Diagram illustrating the placement of a total hip arthroplasty. The femoral head is replaced by a prosthesis with a stem that inserts into the femoral canal. The acetabulum is reamed and a prosthetic cup with a polyethylene liner is inserted

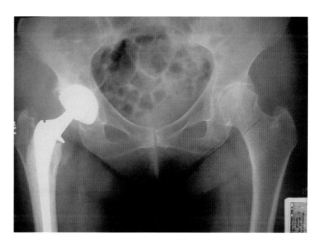

Figure 112 The patient underwent a total hip arthroplasty and was out of bed and walking by postoperative day 2. Patients who undergo total hip or total knee arthroplasties are at an increased risk for deep venous thrombosis. In order to minimize that risk, patients are placed on anticoagulation medication for a period of time surrounding the surgery. Most patients go home on an oral anticoagulant to help protect them from forming a clot

Chapter 5

The knee

ANATOMY

The knee is composed of several distinct articulations including medial and lateral tibiofemoral articulations as well as the patellofemoral articulation. Proper gliding and rolling in the knee are provided through a complex network of ligaments, fibrocartilagenous menisci, and capsular structures. The knee is surrounded by several large muscle groups that also play an important role in its dynamic stability. Anteriorly, the quadriceps inserts onto the patella which is then connected to the tibia through the patellar tendon. This series of muscles and tendons is called the extensor complex. The hamstring muscles run posteriorly from the ischium to the tibia (semi-membranosis, semi-tendinosis) and the fibula (biceps femoris). The major static stability is afforded the knee by the medial and lateral collateral ligaments and the anterior and posterior cruciate ligaments, which serve to restrain valgus and varus forces as well as anterior and posterior forces, respectively.

HISTORY AND PHYSICAL EXAMINATION

If the pain can be localized by the patient, it can often direct the physician toward the pathology. Anterior knee pain that is made worse with climbing stairs and prolonged sitting or squatting should lead the clinician to look for patellofemoral disease. Sharper pain localized to either the posteromedial or posterolateral sides of the knee that is worse with side-to-side movements or twisting can indicate meniscal pathology, and a dull pain exacerbated with changes in the weather and associated with morning stiffness can indicate underlying arthritis. A history of instability or 'giving way' can be due to insufficiency of the anterior cruciate ligament, while less severe episodes can be due to weakness of the quadriceps and patellofemoral problems. Locking is a momentary inability to fully extend the knee and is often associated with displaced meniscal tears or loose bodies.

Physical examination of the knee is performed in a systematic fashion: observation, palpation, range of motion, and provocative maneuvers testing stability are performed. General alignment is assessed as well as gait. In the seated position, the knee is brought through a range of motion and patellar crepitus can be appreciated. The quadriceps and patellar tendons are palpated, as well as the medial and lateral menisci. In the supine position, an effusion can easily be palpated. The active and passive ranges of motion are measured. Pain with hyperflexion is suggestive of meniscal pathology, as is a palpable click over the joint line when the knee is internally and externally rotated (the McMurray test). Patellar mobility is assessed in both the superior–inferior and medial–lateral planes. Apprehension to stress may be a clue to patellar instability. The medial and lateral collateral ligaments are tested both in full extension and in 30° of flexion. The anterior cruciate ligament is tested by attempting to translate the tibia anteriorly with the Lachman test. It can also be tested by trying to reduce an already anteriorly subluxed tibia by bringing the knee from full extension into flexion (the pivot shift test). The posterior cruciate ligament is tested by placing the knee into 90° of flexion and applying a posterior force, then judging the relationship of the tibial tubercle to the femoral condyles (the posterior drawer test).

DIAGNOSTIC STUDIES

Plain radiographs are a necessary component for a complete examination of the knee. They are most helpful in cases of fractures, periosteal reactions, intraosseous lesions, osteoarthritis and in assessing patellofemoral alignment (the merchant view). CT scanning is not as commonly used in the knee now that MRI has become more widely available. MRI is the most useful tool in detecting intra-articular pathology. Ligaments, meniscii, cartilage and the subchondral bone (e.g. in cases of osteochondral lesions and avascular necrosis) can all be readily seen on MRI.

DISORDERS

The most common disorder of the knee are illustrated in Figures 113–137.

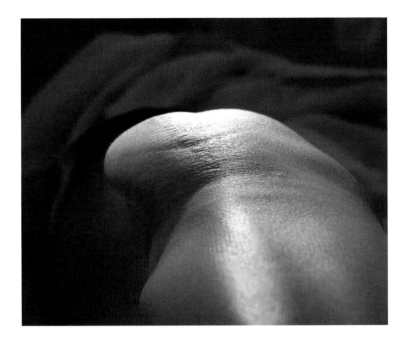

Figure 113 Clinical photograph of a patient who sustained a traumatic lateral patellar dislocation. Most commonly, these injuries reduce themselves before they are seen in the emergency room

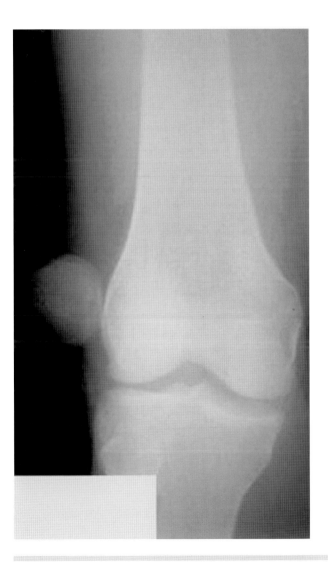

Figure 114 Anteroposterior radiograph of the same patient as in Figure 113

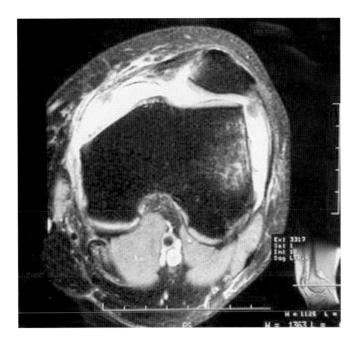

Figure 115 MRI of patients with traumatic patellar dislocation will often reveal a tear of the medial retinacular ligaments and medial patellofemoral ligament. This axial MRI shows the medial patellofemoral ligament to be torn off the adductor tubercle of the femur with a large effusion. Traumatic patellar dislocations are generally treated with temporary immobilization, followed by progressive range of motion and strengthening of the vastus medialis muscle

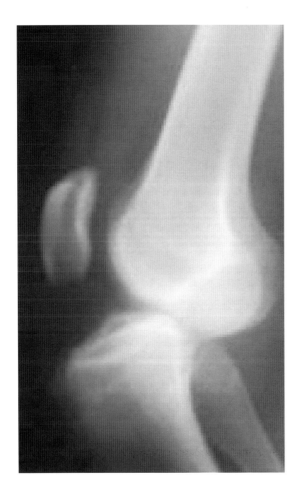

Figure 116 Anteroposterior radiograph of an acute traumatic anterior knee dislocation. Knee dislocations are most commonly high-energy injuries and the physician should maintain a high level of suspicion of associated neurovascular injuries. Careful physical examination and, if necessary, special vascular tests (e.g. angiogram) should be ordered if vascular injury is suspected

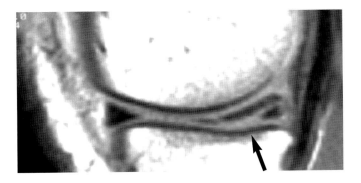

Figure 117 Sagittal MRI of a patient with a posteromedial meniscal tear. Meniscal tears can be traumatic or degenerative and most commonly occur in the posterior horn of the medial meniscus. Tears are demonstrated on MRI based on the presence of fluid that penetrates the meniscus and extends to at least one joint surface

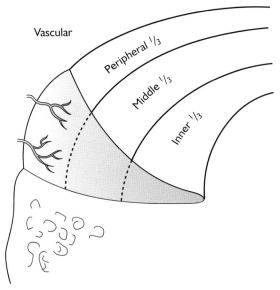

Figure 118 Diagram illustrating the blood supply to the meniscus. The blood supply enters the meniscus from the capsule at the periphery. The meniscus is divided into three zones. The most peripheral third is called the red–red zone because of its proximity to the capsule and its richer blood supply. The middle third is called the red–white zone and has some potential for healing, although less than the more peripheral zone. Tears in this zone are repaired based on the type of tear, the quality of the tissue, and the age of the patient (meniscal repairs are more likely to heal in the presence of a concomitant reconstruction of the anterior cruciate ligament). The innermost third is called the white–white zone and has little to no blood supply and thus is not repaired, but resected instead

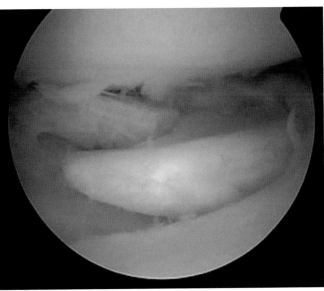

Figure 119 Arthroscopic photograph of a medial meniscal tear. The tear was debrided to alleviate the patient's symptoms of pain and catching

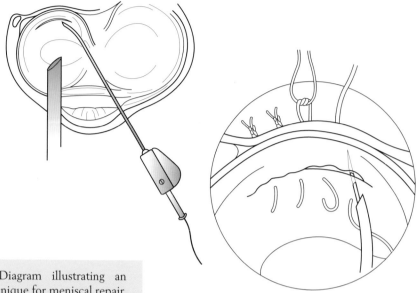

Figure 120 Diagram illustrating an inside-out technique for meniscal repair. Depending upon the location, the surgeon may wish to use an outside-in, an inside-out, or an all-inside technique to repair the meniscus

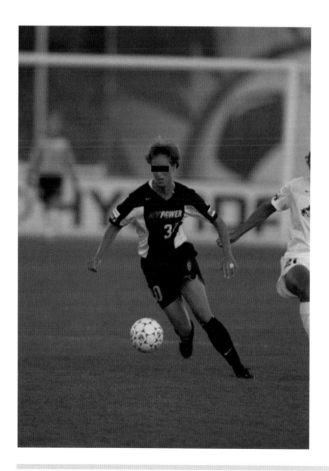

Figure 121 Photograph of a female soccer player illustrating the valgus twisting motion that is the most commonly responsible mechanism for non-contact injury to the anterior cruciate ligament (ACL). ACL injuries are much more common in the female athlete than in the male athlete. Many hypotheses have been proposed as to why females are at an increased risk including notch-size, hormonal influence, alignment, and muscle imbalances. No one theory has been proven and significant research continues in this interesting area

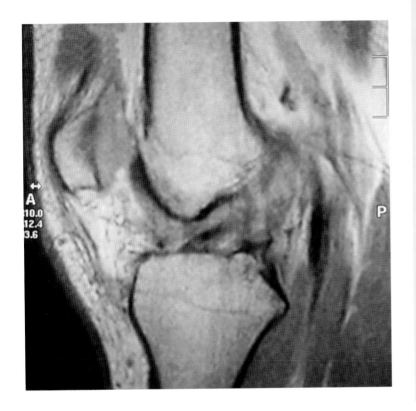

Figure 122 T1-weighted sagittal oblique magnetic resonance image of the intercondylar notch of the knee in a 17-year-old young man who was playing soccer and sustained a twisting non-contact injury to his knee. He reported hearing a 'pop' and feeling his knee give way. He developed a rapid effusion and said that his knee had been giving away since the injury. This image demonstrates a complete tear of the anterior cruciate ligament (ACL) at its femoral origin. The tibial insertion remains attached. ACL reconstructions are generally recommended in young active patients who wish to continue their active lifestyle and who are experiencing instability. Certain sports are much more ACL-dependent than others: basketball, soccer, lacrosse, and elite-level tennis all require a significant amount of cutting and pivoting. Patients who elect not to undergo ACL reconstruction and have continued instability episodes with subluxations are more likely to tear their meniscus than those whose knees are stable

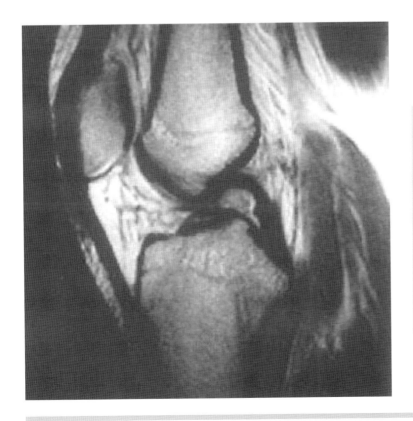

Figure 123 Sagittal oblique MRI through the intercondylar notch. The posterior cruciate ligament (PCL) is usually seen on MRI just medial to the anterior cruciate ligament (ACL). The PCL runs from the medial femoral condyle to the posterior proximal tibia and is responsible for restraining posterior tibial translation. The PCL is much less commonly injured than the ACL. The mechanism of injury is usually a fall onto a flexed knee or a dashboard injury in a motor vehicle accident

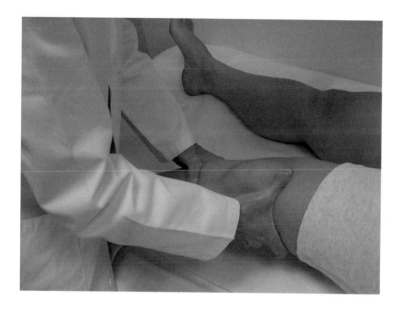

Figure 124 The Lachman examination is the most sensitive maneuver to test for competency of the anterior cruciate ligament. One hand is used to stabilize the femur and the other is used to pull the tibia anteriorly. The non-injured knee should always be examined first in order to determine physiological laxity. The injured knee is flexed to approximately 30° and an anterior force is applied. A positive test is graded on both the amount of anterior translation as well as the sensation of a firm or soft endpoint

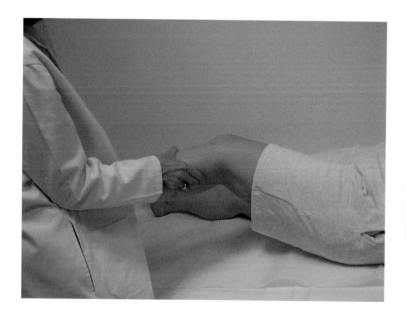

Figure 125 The Pivot shift test is another test used to examine for insufficiency of the anterior cruciate ligament (ACL). The knee is brought from full extension (where the tibia is subluxed anteriorly on the femur) into 30° of flexion, the tibia held in slight internal rotation. When the knee is flexed, the tibia will reduce posteriorly on the femur. This can be both sensed and visualized by the examiner

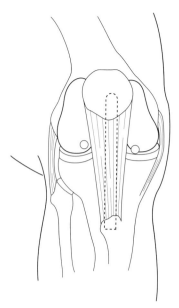

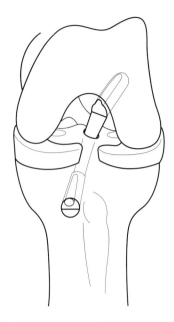

Figure 126 Diagram illustrating the graft harvest site most commonly used. Bone–patellar tendon–bone is the most common graft used to reconstruct the anterior cruciate ligament. There are many other graft sources available to the physician and the decisions on which one to use is based on many factors including the patient's history and the surgeon's preference

Figure 127 The final anterior cruciate ligament reconstruction is illustrated in this diagram. Drill holes are created under arthroscopic visualization, on the posterior wall of the lateral femoral condyle as well as on the medial side of the anterior tibia. The graft is then brought through the drill holes and secured on the femoral side. Next, tension is placed on the graft as the knee is brought through a range of motion to remove any creep and the tibial side of the graft is secured

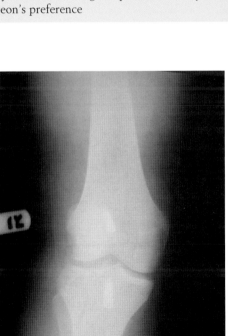

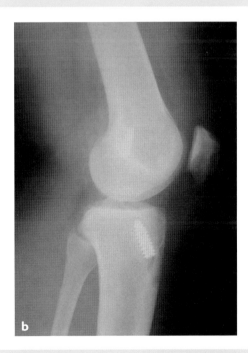

Figure 128 Anteroposterior (a) and lateral (b) radiographs of a patient who underwent anterior cruciate ligament reconstruction with bone tendon–bone autograft. The graft was secured on both the femur and the tibia with metal interference screws. Radiographs can provide useful information on tunnel placement and bone plug healing

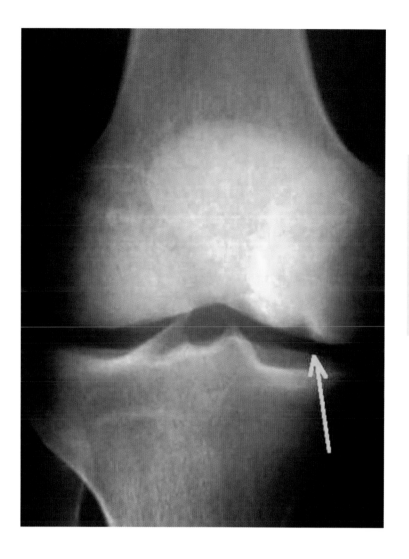

Figure 129 Anteroposterior radiograph of a patient with an osteochondritis dessicans (OCD) lesion. The lesion is most commonly seen on the lateral aspect of the medial femoral condyle, as in this radiograph. This patient's symptoms included pain and locking of the knee with sports. The lesion is often seen in children with open growth plates, and these patients have the best prognosis

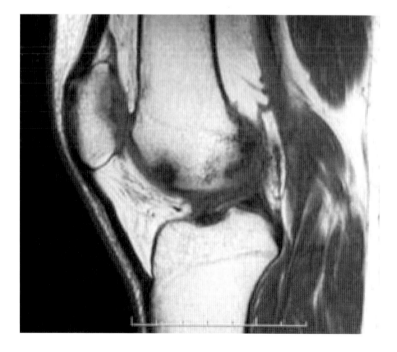

Figure 130 Sagittal oblique T1-weighted MRI demonstrating the appearance of an osteochondritis dessicans lesion. In this patient, the cartilage has not yet separated from the underlying bone

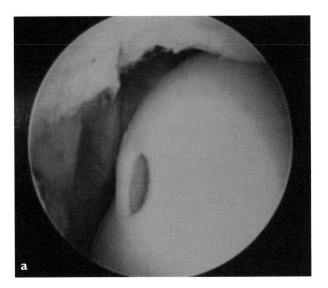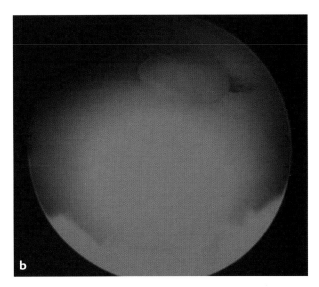

Figure 131 In older patients with focal chondral defects (as in osteochondritis dessicans lesion), there are several options as to how and with what to fill the defect. Bone marrow stimulation techniques, such as microfracture and drilling, allow filling of the defect with fibrocartilage. Techniques such as osteochondral autograft transplantation (OATS) take articular cartilage plugs from non-weight-bearing regions (a) of the knee and use these plugs to fill the traumatic defect (b)

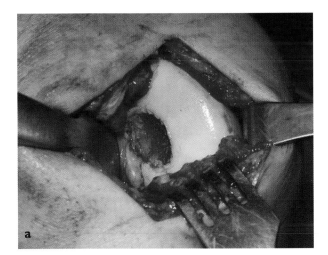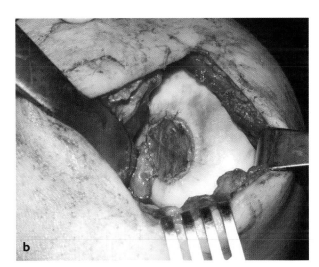

Figure 132 Another option for treating focal cartilage defects (a) is autologous chondrocyte implantation (ACI). This method is fairly new and involves taking a small biopsy of healthy cartilage (arthroscopically) and growing the chondrocytes *ex vivo* in a laboratory. The patient is then brought back to the operating room and the chondrocytes are injected into the cartilage defect (b) and held in place with a periosteal flap

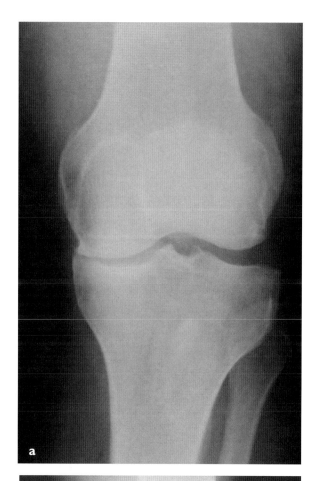

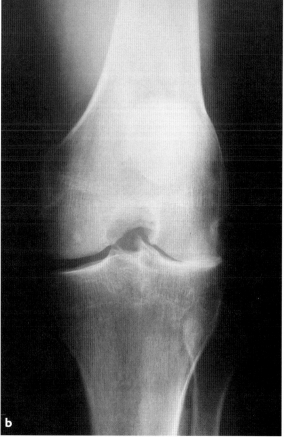

Figure 133 Anteroposterior radiographs of patients with unicompartmental osteoarthritis of the medial (a) and lateral (b) compartments. In younger more active patients with unicompartmental disease, total knee arthroplasty and unicompartmental arthroplasty are not very good options due to the high rates of wear which necessitate revision surgery. High tibial osteotomies correct the malalignment and transfer the weight-bearing forces to the opposite compartment with healthier cartilage. The benefit of the osteotomy versus an arthroplasty is that there is no risk of prosthetic wear, and patients can go back to their active lifestyles

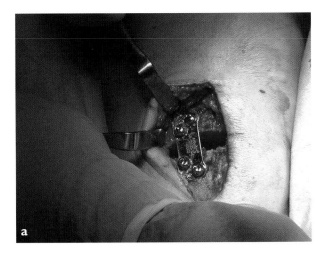

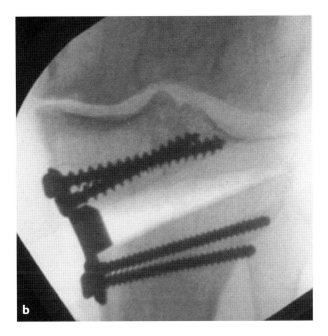

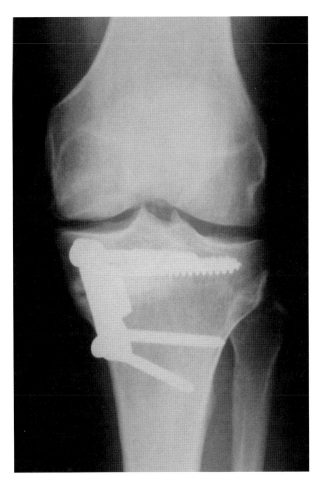

Figure 135   Postoperative anteroposterior radiograph of a patient who underwent a high-tibial opening wedge osteotomy. The radiograph demonstrates a significant improvement in the alignment of the knee and good healing of the bone graft

Figure 134   Intraoperative photograph (a) and fluoroscopy (b) of a medial opening wedge osteotomy for medial compartment arthritis. the amount of opening is calculated pre-operatively by the number of degrees needed for correction of the malalignment. Approximately 1 mm of opening is needed for every degree of correction desired

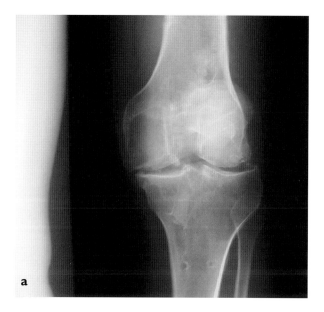

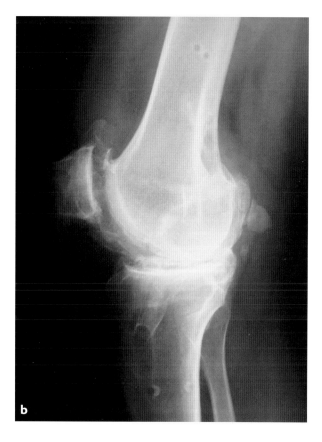

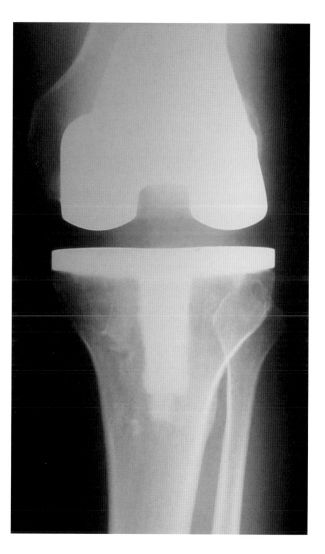

Figure 137 Anteroposterior radiograph of the same patient after total knee replacement. These are very successful in relieving pain and improving function. Patients are encouraged to start ambulating on postoperative day 1 or 2 in order to minimize the risk of deep venous thrombosis and pulmonary embolus. In addition to the rapid mobilization, patients are fitted with pneumatic devices for the feet to keep the blood circulating and are anticoagulated to prevent the formation of a clot

Figure 136 Anteroposterior (a) and lateral (b) radiographs of a patient with advanced tricompartmental degenerative joint disease

Chapter 6

The foot and ankle

ANATOMY

The foot is generally divided into three regions: the forefoot, mid-foot, and hindfoot. The forefoot is made up of the five metatarsals and 14 phalanges. The mid-foot consists of the five tarsal bones, and the hindfoot contains the calcaneus and the talus. The talus is unique in that about 60–70% of its surface is covered with articular cartilage and it has no musculotendinous attachments. The ankle is basically a hinge joint, with the talus held firmly between the two malleoli (tibial and fibular) to create the mortisse joint. The subtalar joint is the talocalcaneal joint and is responsible for inversion and eversion. Chopart's joint is composed of the talonavicular and calcaneocuboid joints and is the anatomic junction of the hindfoot and mid-foot. Lisfranc's joints are the tarsal–metatarsal articulations. It is through the Lisfranc joints that much of the supination and pronation occur.

The ligamentous network about the foot and ankle provides significant stability. Medially, the deltoid ligament is a fan-shaped structure consisting of superficial and deep layers. Laterally, the ankle is stabilized by three ligaments: the anterior talofibular ligament, posterior talofibular ligament, and calcaneofibular ligament. Plantar muscles covered with fascia originate off the calcaneus and are frequently responsible for plantar foot pain.

HISTORY AND PHYSICAL EXAMINATION

Pain is again the predominant presenting symptom for which patients seek evaluation. It is important to characterize the pain as to its location, its character, what makes it better or worse and its relationship to walking and/or shoes. Physical examination in this region should consist not only of the foot, but the shoe as well. It can be very helpful to examine the sole of the shoe to characterize abnormal wear patterns that might suggest an abnormal gait pattern. The foot should be inspected both standing and sitting. With standing, the heel should be central, the toes straight, and the arch should be maintained. While sitting, the foot should be supple with a good range of motion in all joints. The skin should be inspected for areas of increased pressure reflected as corns or calluses. Finally, a thorough neurovascular examination should be completed. Deformities such as bunions and hammer toes are frequently visible on the initial examination.

DIAGNOSTIC STUDIES

Plain radiographs, although helpful, are somewhat limited in the foot and ankle because the number and position of the joints make visualization difficult. Computerized tomography is especially valuable in assessing the subtalar and mid-foot joints. Tarsal coalitions, fractures of the os calcis and talus as well as mid-foot fracture dislocations (Lisfranc injuries) are seen particularly well with this technique. MRI is finding broader indications in the foot and ankle. Specifically, the diagnoses of stress fractures and enthesopathies such as posterior tibial tendon insufficiency are much easier seen with MRI than with other modalities.

In the diabetic foot, Doppler evaluation for the diagnosis of vascular insufficiency is an invaluable tool. Evaluation of blood flow can often assist in the decisions regarding treatment in these patients.

DISORDERS

The most common disorders about the foot and ankle are illustrated in Figures 138–171.

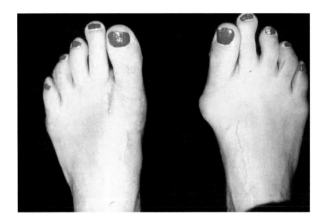

Figure 138 Photograph of a patient with bilateral hallux valgus. She underwent correction of the left hallux valgus approximately 6 months previously. The incision between the first and second metatarsals is used to release the adductor halucis

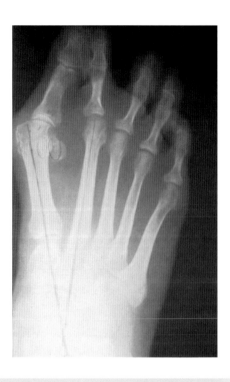

Figure 140 Pre-operative radiograph of a patient with a hallux valgus deformity. The intermetatarsal angle is increased, the metarsal head is left uncovered by the subluxation of the first metatarsal–phalangeal joint, and the sesmoids are dislocated laterally

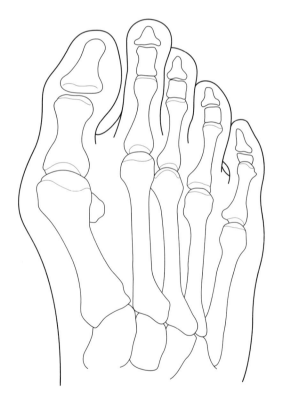

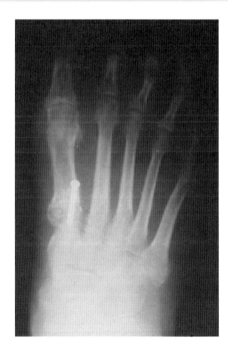

Figure 139 Diagram illustrating the patho-anatomy of hallux valgus. There are a wide variety of surgical osteotomies that can be used to correct hallux valgus. The choice of osteotomy depends both on the severity of the deformity and the congruity or incongruity of the meta-tarsal–phalangeal joint

Figure 141 Postoperative radiograph of the same patient as in Figure 140 after surgical correction with a proximal osteotomy of the first metatarsal

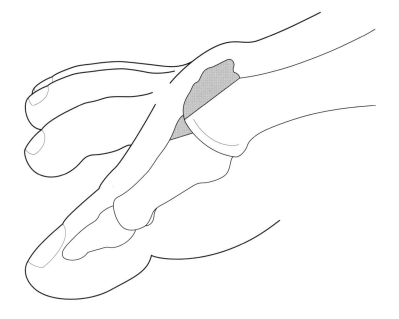

Figure 142 Diagram illustrating the dorsal osteophyte associated with hallux rigidus. Hallux rigidus is a condition resulting in limited range of motion at the metatarsal–phalangeal joint of the great toe. The cause of hallux rigidus is unclear. It may result from a single traumatic event that causes injury to the dorsal cartilage of the meta-tarsal–phalangeal joint, or from degener-ative arthritis of the first meta-tarsal–phalangeal joint with resulting synovitis and osteophyte proliferation

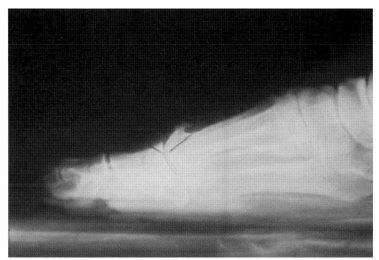

Figure 143 Lateral radiograph of the foot demonstrating the dorsal osteo-phyte commonly seen in hallux rigidus

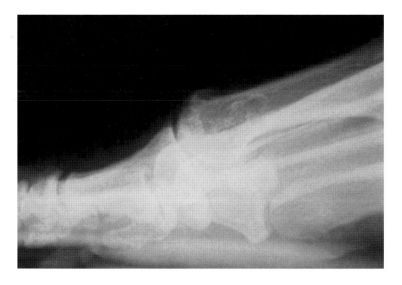

Figure 144 Postoperative radiograph of the same patient after treatment of hallux rigidus by removal of the dorsal osteophytes

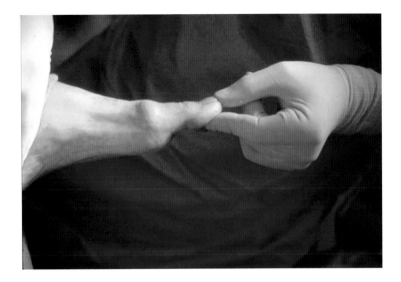

Figure 145 Clinical photograph of the limited motion (specifically dorsiflexion) caused by hallux rigidus

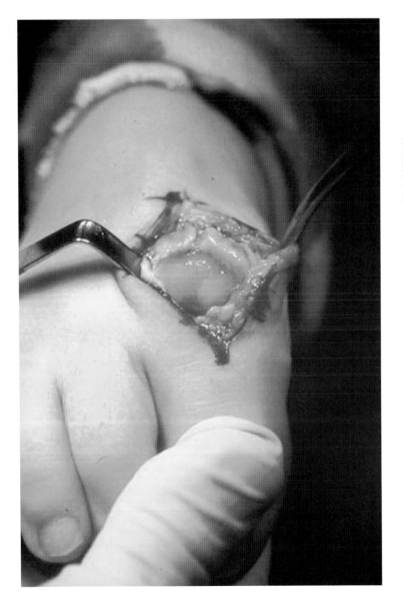

Figure 146 Intraoperative photograph of the dorsal osteophytes on the distal metatarsal head

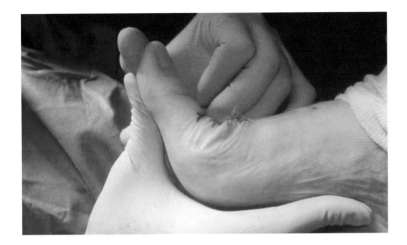

Figure 147 Clinical postoperative photograph of the dorsiflexion regained after removal of the osteophytes

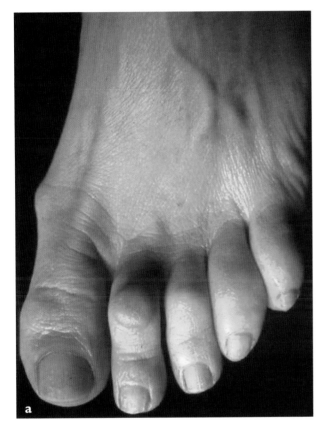

Figure 148 Clinical photographs (frontal (a) and lateral (b)) of hammer-toe deformities of the second toe with an associated corn over the proximal interphalangeal joint (PIP). A hammer-toe is a flexion deformity of the PIP, usually seen with a corresponding extension posture of the metatarsal–phalangeal joint of the same toe. The deformity may be fixed or flexible

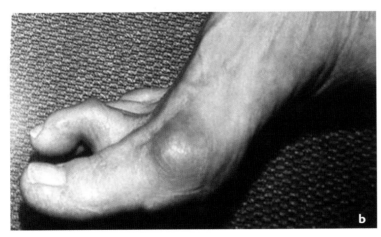

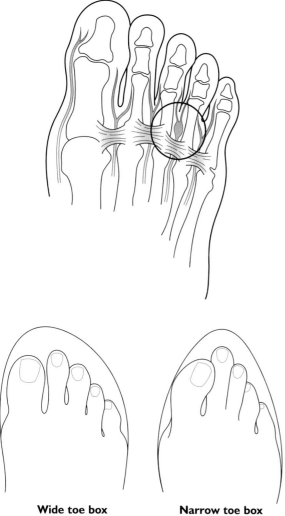

Figure 149 Diagram illustrating the pathoanatomy of an intermetatarsal digital neuroma (Morton's neuroma)

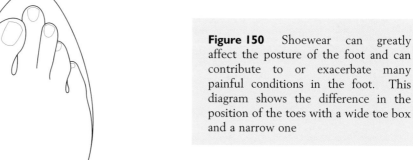

Wide toe box   **Narrow toe box**

Figure 150 Shoewear can greatly affect the posture of the foot and can contribute to or exacerbate many painful conditions in the foot. This diagram shows the difference in the position of the toes with a wide toe box and a narrow one

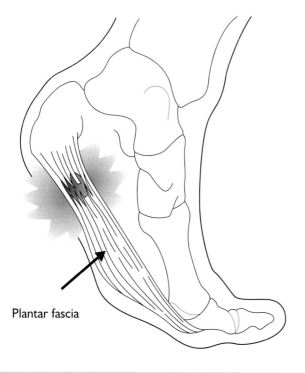

Plantar fascia

Figure 151 Diagram illustrating the painful condition of plantar fasciitis. The plantar fascia originates from the anteromedial plantar aspect of the calcaneal tuberosity and inserts across the metatarsal–phalangeal joints. One possible theory as to why people develop plantar foot pain is the so-called windlass mechanism, the tightening of the fascia with dorsiflexion of the toes, causing traction on the origin of the plantar fascia

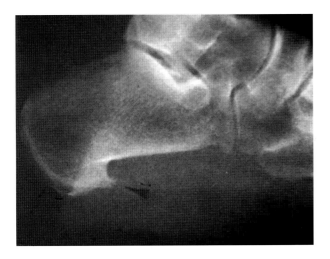

Figure 152 Radiograph of a calcaneal spur. Radiographs reveal a calcaneal spur in about 50% of patients with plantar fascia symptoms, but the significance of this finding is uncertain

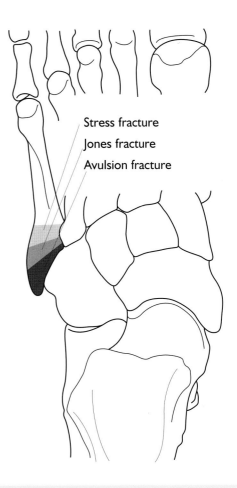

Stress fracture
Jones fracture
Avulsion fracture

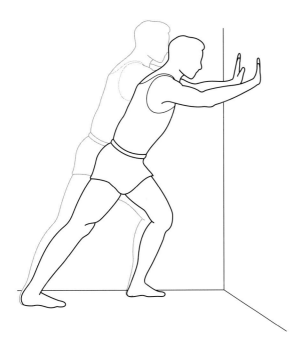

Figure 153 The treatment of patients with plantar fasciitis consists of a combination of oral non-steroidal anti-inflammatory medications, heel cups, night splints and physical therapy consisting of Achilles tendon stretches. Most patients respond favorably to non-operative treatment of this condition

Figure 154 Diagram illustrating the most common sites for 5th metatarsal fractures. The varying blood supply to the bone in this region means that the treatment of these fractures differs depending on their location, despite their close proximity to one another. Fracture of the most proximal portion of the 5th metatarsal is usually an avulsion injury caused by inversion to the plantar flexed foot. This fracture is treated with a short leg walking cast and, although some fractures may go on to non-union, they are generally not painful and, if necessary can be treated with excision of the fragment. The fractures that occur in the metaphyseal–diaphyseal and the diaphyseal regions are usually of the acute-on-chronic variety, with the patient having a prodromal period of pain and/or radiographic evidence of sclerosis. These are regions of poor vascularity and thus should be treated with cast immobilization and non-weight-bearing for at least 6 weeks. In elite athletes or patients who cannot be treated by non-weight-bearing, consideration should be given to intramedullary screw fixation

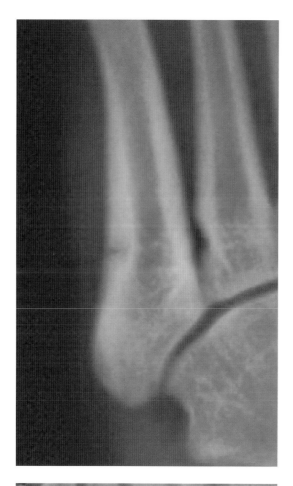

Figure 155   Anteroposterior radiograph of an elite high-school basketball player with a stress fracture at the base of the fifth metatarsal

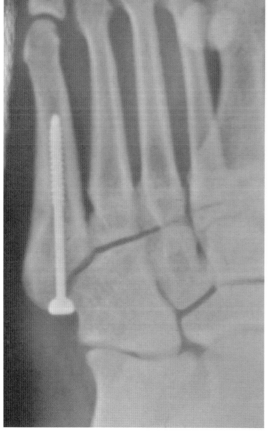

Figure 156   This player was treated with intramedullary screw fixation to allow for early weight-bearing and a faster return to play

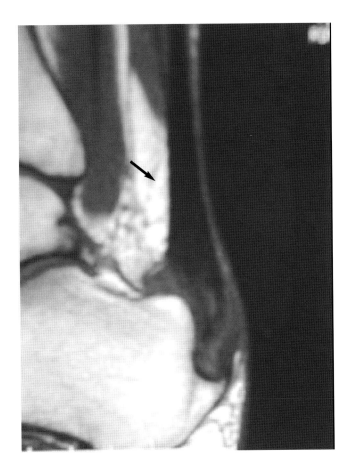

Figure 157 Sagittal MRI of a patient with chronic Achilles tendinosis. The tendinosis usually occurs 3–4 cm proximal to the insertion of the tendon as a tender, thickened and sometimes bulbous mass

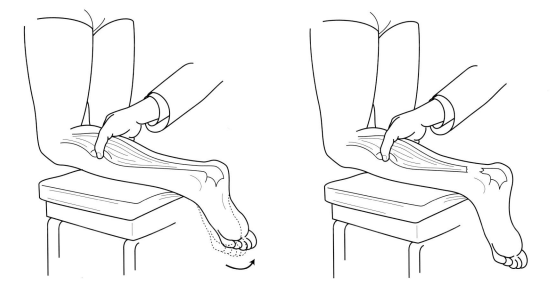

Figure 158 Achilles tendon rupture is usually the result of a forceful eccentric contraction of the gastrocnemius–soleus complex and most commonly occurs during sports-related activities. The majority of these injuries occur in patients in their 3rd and 4th decades. The Thompson test is positive in the presence of an Achilles rupture. With the patient prone and the knee flexed, the gastrocnemius–soleus complex is squeezed by the examiner while close attention is payed to the posture of the foot. If the foot plantar flexes with this maneuver, then the Achilles tendon is intact. If the foot remains flaccid, then an Achilles tendon rupture should be suspected

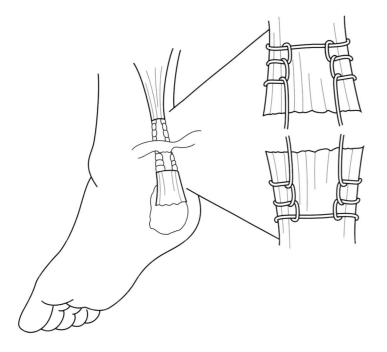

Figure 159 Diagram illustrating the authors' preferred method of tendon repair. The majority of tendon ruptures occur in the middle third of the tendon. A medial skin incision is made and the ends of the tendon are freshened. A strong non-absorbable suture is placed in both the proximal and distal ends in a krackow fashion (as illustrated); the ends of the tendon are then approximated and the sutures are tied

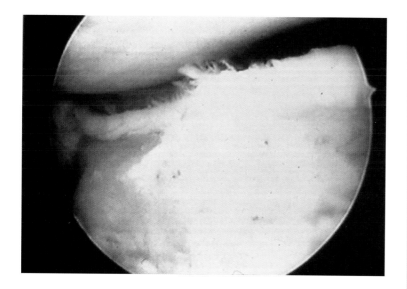

Figure 160 Arthroscopic photograph of the tibio–talar joint with significant arthritis. Cartilage loss can be focal, as is the case with traumatic osteochondral injuries, or global, such as in patients with previous intra-articular fractures that have gone on to develop arthritis. Focal cartilage lesions are difficult to treat. Marrow stimulation techniques (such as drilling or micro-fracture) are often employed to promote filling of the defect with fibrocartilage in the hope of relieving the patient's symptoms. In cases of global arthritis, ankle fusion and total ankle arthroplasty are the most common surgical options. As technology improves, total ankle arthroplasty is becoming a more realistic option; however, ankle fusion remains the most common form of treatment for advanced and debilitating ankle arthritis

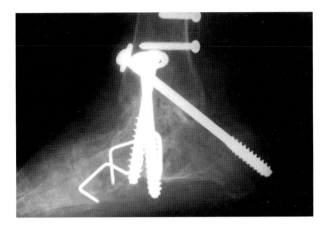

Figure 161   Lateral radiograph of an ankle fusion

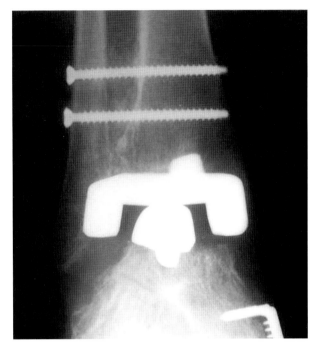

Figure 163   Anteroposterior radiograph of a total ankle arthroplasty

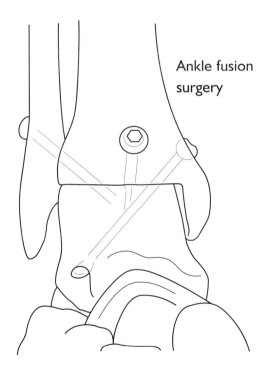

Figure 162   Diagram of a tibio–talar fusion

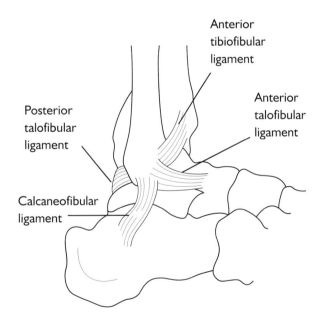

Figure 164   Diagram of the lateral side of the ankle illustrating the ligaments most commonly injured in an inversion ankle sprain. The anterior talofibular ligament is the most commonly injured followed by the calcaneo-fibular ligament

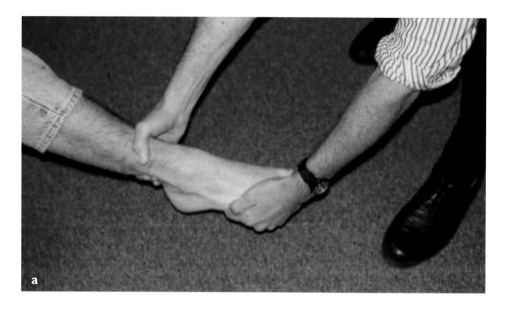

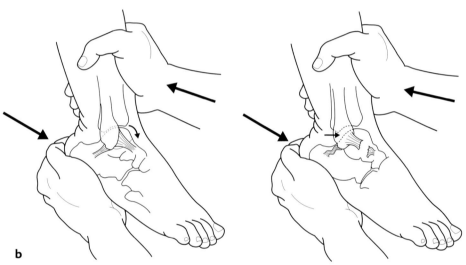

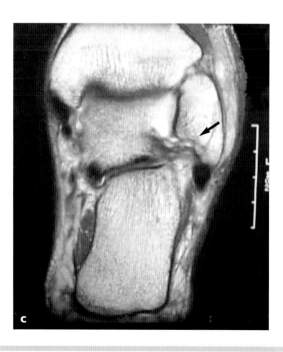

Figure 165 Clinical (a) and diagrammatic (b) illustrations of the anterior drawer test used to elicit ligamentous laxity and ankle instability. The injured or symptomatic side is tested and compared to the contralateral side for control. In cases of chronic instability with repeated ankle ligament injury, the talus can be anteriorly displaced from the tibia without restraint from the anterior talofibular ligament (ATFL). The coronal MRI (c) demonstrates increased signal and edema in the AFTL. The fibers of the ATFL look wavy, probably caused by multiple injuries to that ligament

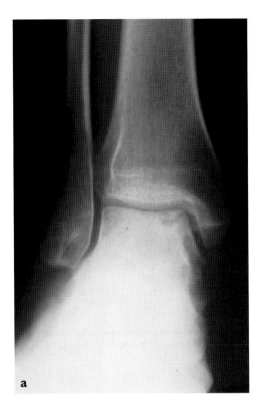

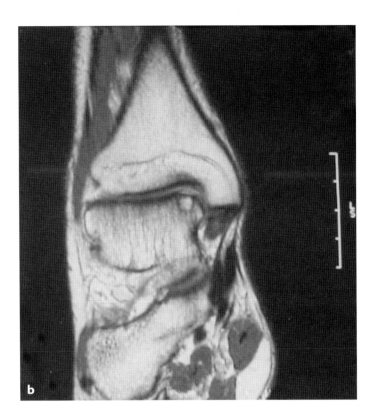

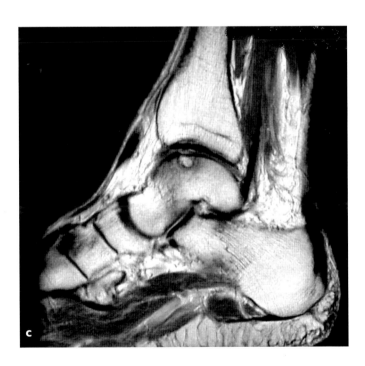

Figure 166 Anteroposterior radiograph (a) and coronal (b) and sagittal oblique (c) MR images demonstrating an anteromedial osteochondritis dessicans lesion of the talar dome. This 43-year-old marathoner had no history of injury, but had worsening pain and grinding with dorsiflexion and plantar flexion, limiting him from running

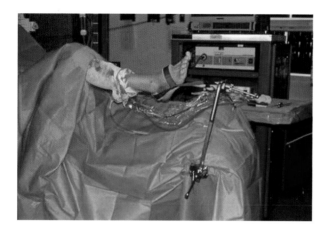

Figure 167 Ankle arthroscopy is performed with the patient placed in the supine position. The symptomatic ankle is prepped out and a sterile traction strap is placed distally so as not to obscure portal placement. Traction is used to fascilitate arthroscopic visualization

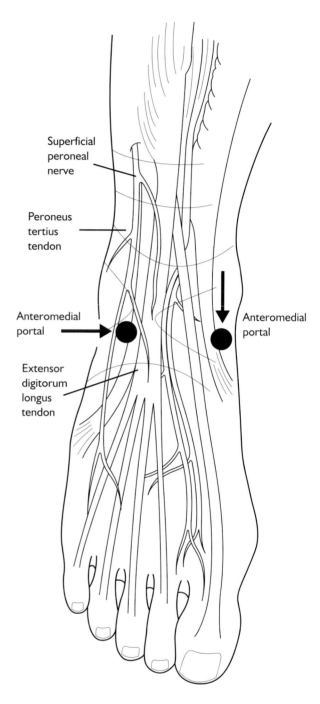

Figure 169 Diagram illustrating the most commonly used anteromedial and anterolateral portals. The anterolateral portal is created just lateral to the peroneus tertius, making sure to avoid the superficial branch of the peroneal nerve. The anteromedial portal is created medial to the anterior tibialis tendon. Injury to the saphenous nerve is avoided by staying close to the tendon and not placing the portal too far medially

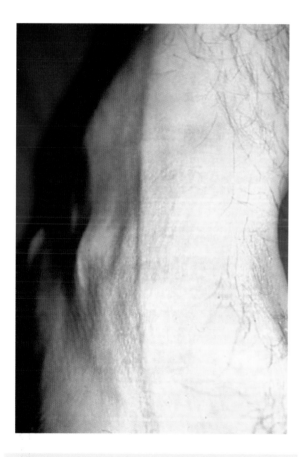

Figure 168 The superficial peroneal nerve is readily identified on the lateral side of the ankle by plantar flexion and inversion, and should be marked prior to the creation of the portals to avoid injury

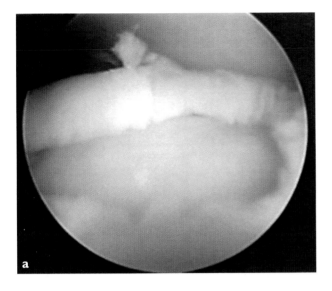

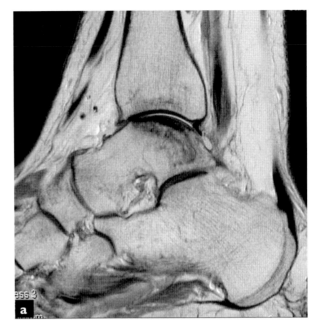

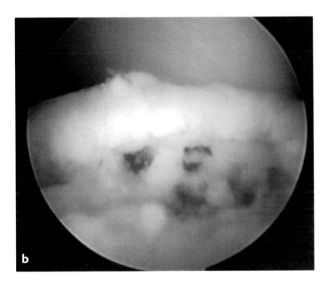

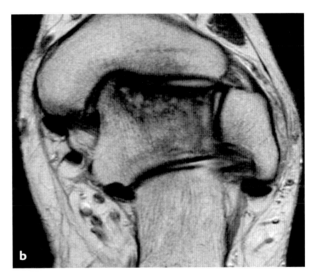

Figure 170 Arthroscopic photographs taken of the same patient with an osteochondritis dessicans lesion. The lesion was peeled away from the bone causing the patient's symptoms of grinding and locking.   The cartilage was unstable and thus debrided (a) to leave this stable rim surrounding the defect. Next the defect was picked with a sharp awl to bring in capillary blood flow and stimulate fibro-cartilage ingrowth into the defect (b). The patient was non-weight-bearing for 6 weeks after this proce-dure to allow the fibrocartilage to fill in. Aggressive range of motion exercises were started immediately to prevent stiffness

Figure 171 Sagittal (a) and coronal (b) MRIs demonstrating a patient who went on to develop avascular necrosis of the talar dome after sustaining a minimally displaced fracture several years ago. The blood supply to the talus is very tenuous, much like that to the scaphoid, and thus fractures in this bone should be treated aggressively and followed closely to prevent complications such as avascular necrosis

Chapter 7

Pediatrics

The field of pediatric orthopedics is deserving of an atlas all to itself. However, this Atlas illustrates many of the most common disorders.

The pediatric patient is often unable to give a detailed history and so the clinician must rely on the parent history, physical examination, imaging studies and sometimes laboratory studies to aid in the diagnosis and treatment.

PHYSICAL EXAMINATION

The physical examination should consist of inspection of the whole body since subtleties such as skin lesions (café au lait spots in congenital scoliosis) and skin creases (asymmetric creases in the thigh with developmental dysplasia of the hip) can often help to guide the surgeon to the correct diagnosis. The range of motion of the joints should be checked as well as the posture or angulation of the extremities. The surgeon must know the changes in joint angulation (i.e. varus and valgus) that occur with growth in order to distinguish physiological angulation from pathological angulation (i.e. Blount's syndrome).

DIAGNOSTIC STUDIES

Simple radiographs are sometimes all that is needed to confirm a diagnosis. For example, the presence of multiple long bone fractures in various stages of healing may provide clues to an abusive environment. Since open physes and variable ossification can make radiographic interpretation difficult, it is often helpful to have symptomatic and contralateral asymptomatic structures evaluated radiographically.

The introduction of more advanced imaging capabilities, such as MRI, positron emission testing (PET), and ultrasound have enhanced our ability to make early diagnoses (as early as *in utero*) of pediatric disorders and to change outcomes based on early intervention. MRI has helped to differentiate idiopathic scoliosis from congenital scoliosis, as well as to guide the preoperative planning. PET scanning has become a helpful tool in the diagnosis of spondylolisthesis, and ultrasound is very popular for assessing and monitoring hip reduction in cases of developmental hip dysplasia.

DISORDERS

Pediatric orthopedic disorders are illustrated in Figures 172–204.

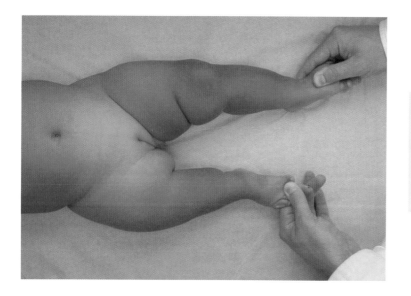

Figure 172 Asymmetric gluteal folds are one of the signs of possible developmental dysplasia of the hip. This child's right leg is shorter and the folds are asymmetric; further testing should be carried out to determine the underlying pathology

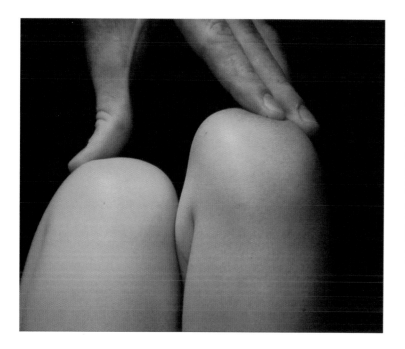

Figure 173 The Galeazzi sign is demonstrated with both feet and knees together; if the heights of the knees are different, a foreshortened limb is indicated. Another cause of a positive Galeazzi test besides developmental dysplasia of the hip (DDH) is a congenitally short femur. Both the gluteal folds and the Galeazzi tests will be negative in patients with bilateral DDH and this diagnosis should be carefully excluded

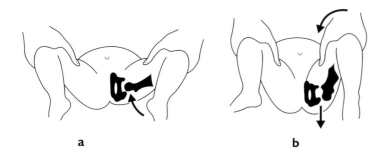

a   b

Figure 174 The most reliable tests on physical examination are the Ortolani and Barlow tests. This diagram illustrates these provocative maneuvers. In the Ortolani test (a), the femur is elevated and abducted and a previously dislocated hip is reduced with a palpable click. The Barlow test (b) consists of adduction and depression of the femur, which will dislocate a dislocatable hip

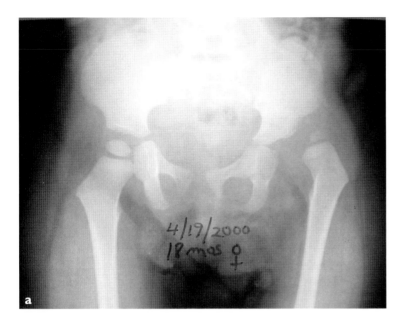

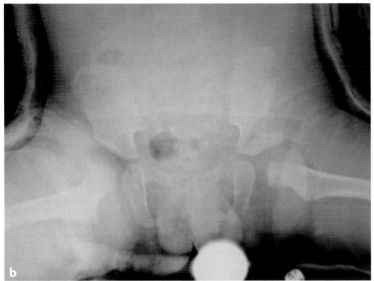

Figure 175 Anteroposterior radiographs of a dislocated hip in developmental dysplasia of the hip (DDH) (a) and of the patient in the abducted and externally rotated position (b) with the hip reduced. DDH represents an abnormal development of the hip secondary to both capsular laxity as well as mechanical factors such as intrauterine position. DDH is more likely in females, first-born children, and breech positioning

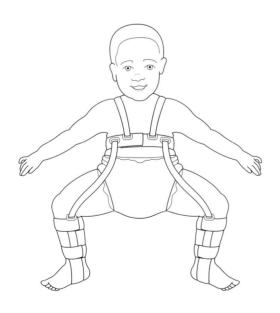

Figure 176 A Pavlik harness is used in infants to maintain the hip in the reduced position. Ultrasound is a very useful tool for follow-up checks to ensure that the hip reduction is maintained

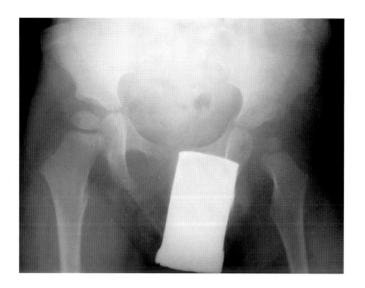

Figure 177 After successful reduction, the femoral head and acetabulum start to develop in a more normal fashion. Depending on the duration of the dislocation, the femoral head may appear smaller and somewhat delayed in development on subsequent radiographs as is seen in this anteroposterior radiograph

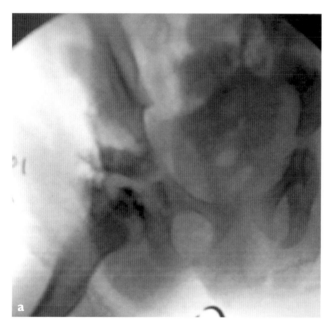

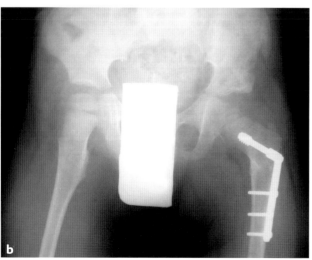

Figure 178 Osteotomies may be required for persistent instability, progressive femoral head subluxation after reduction, or acetabular dysplasia. Pelvic osteotomies, such as the one shown here (a), can provide better femoral head coverage and better stability to the dysplastic hip. Varus osteotomies of the femur (VDRO) (b) are used to correct marked anteversion or coxa valga and are generally used in children under 4 years of age

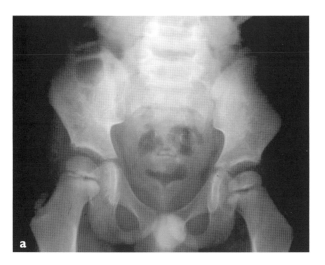
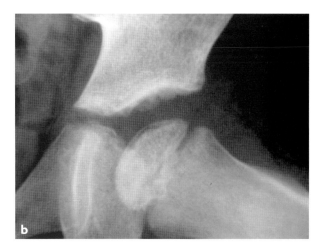

Figure 179 Anteroposterior (a) and lateral (b) radiographs of a patient with Legg–Calve–Perthes (LCP). LCP is a deformity of the femoral head resulting from a vascular insult. The proximal femoral epiphyses undergoes osteonecrosis with resultant pain and a limp. LCP is most commonly seen in young boys between 4 and 8 years old and the incidence is increased with a positive family history. Prognosis is based upon the age at presentation. The younger the patient, the better the prognosis because the epiphysis has more time to revascularize and remodel after the insult. Patients are generally treated symptomatically with non-steroidal anti-inflammatories and partial weight-bearing, and the radiographs are followed to ensure that the femoral head remains spherical

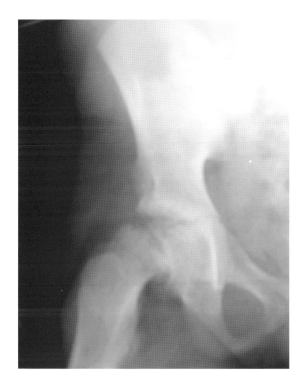

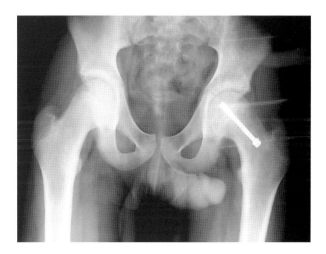

Figure 181 Anteroposterior radiograph of another patient with a slipped capital femoral epiphyses who underwent an in situ pinning to prevent further slippage of the epiphysis

Figure 180 Anteroposterior radiograph demonstrating a slipped capital femoral epiphysis (SCFE). This is a slip through the hypertrophic zone of the proximal femoral epiphysis. It has a high association with male sex, obesity and African–American descent

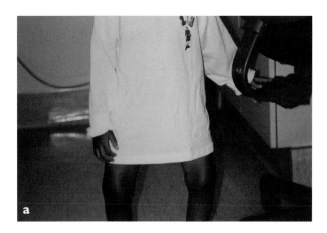
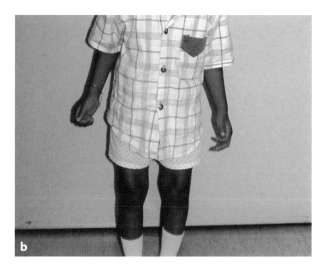

Figure 182 Photograph (a) of a young boy brought into the doctor's office at 20 months for bowed legs. Normally, young children go from genu varum to genu valgum by age 2½ years and progress to more normal physiological valgus by age 4 years. The same patient is pictured at 4½ years old with a near normal alignment of the lower extremities (b). Parents should be reassured that this change is a normal part of the child's development

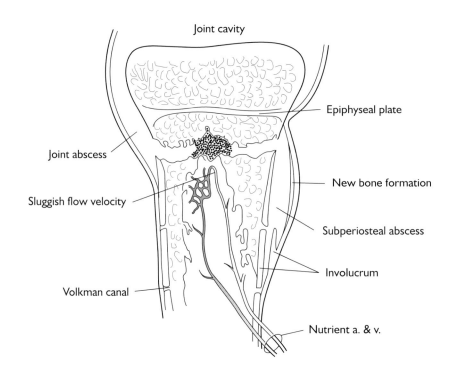

Figure 183 Diagram of the metaphyseal blood flow in pediatric patients. Osteomyelitis is much more common in children because of this unique blood flow. The infection is usually spread hematogenously to the bony metaphysis and, because the blood flow is sluggish where the arterioles bend around the physis, the organisms have a chance to take hold and form a bone abscess

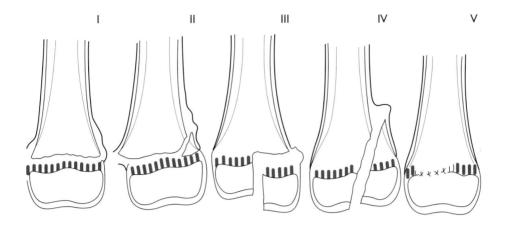

Figure 184 Pediatric fractures are classified and treated differently from adult trauma because of the numerous growth plates and apophyses. The Salter–Harris classification is used to guide both treatment and prognosis based upon the fracture's relationship to the growth plate. A type I fracture is a non-displaced injury through the growth plate, a type II fracture extends from the growth plate proximally into the metaphysis, a type III fracture extends from the growth plate distally to the articular surface, a type IV fracture extends from the metaphysis through the growth plate and to the articular surface and, finally, a type V fracture is a compression fracture which can severely damage the growth plate. All growth plate injuries can lead to growth arrest and asymmetry and the parents should always be advised of this

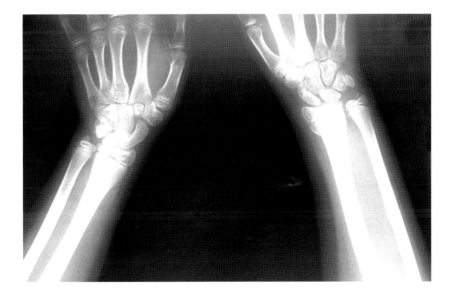

Figure 185 Comparison radiographs are very important in children because the growth plates can often look like fracture lines and comparison with the non-injured side helps to determine the true nature of the injury

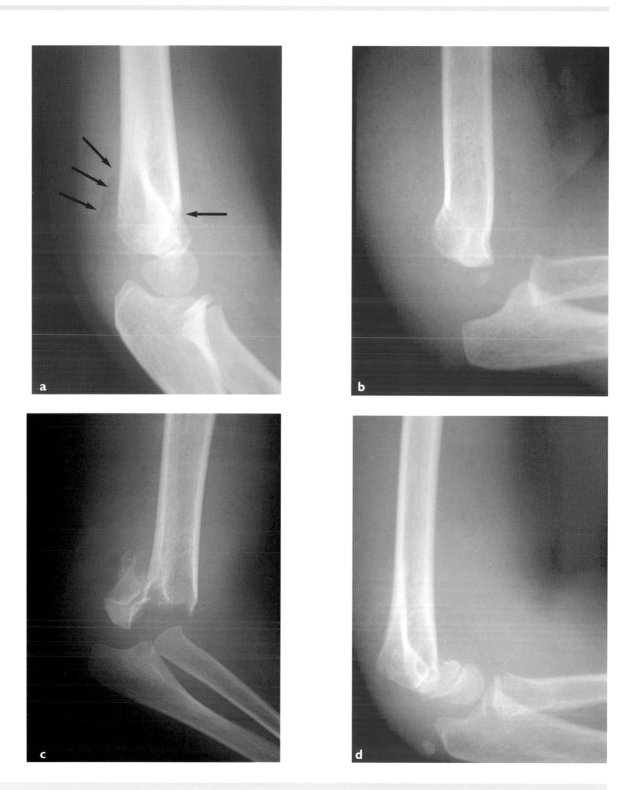

Figure 186   Elbow fractures are some of the most common pediatric injuries seen in the orthopedic clinic and emergency room. Supracondylar fractures are by far the most common elbow fractures seen in children. Two types of supracondylar fractures are seen, depending on the mechanism of injury. More than 90% of supracondylar fractures are of the extension type, with the flexion type as a far second. The extension type is further divided, based on the amount of displacement seen. Type I (a) is a non-displaced fracture; often the fracture line is not even appreciated on the lateral radiograph. Instead, elevation of the posterior fat pad helps to guide the clinician to this diagnosis. Type II fractures (b) are displaced with the posterior cortex remaining intact and serving as a hinge. Type III (c) fractures are completely displaced. The less common flexion type (d) of fracture has a high incidence of neurovascular injury associated with it

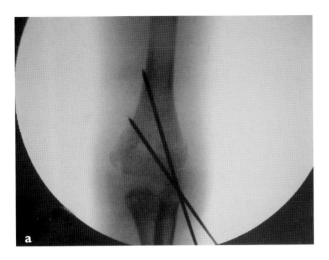
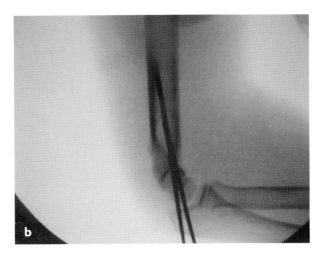

Figure 187 Intraoperative fluoroscopic anteroposterior (a) and lateral (b) views of a reduced and pinned supra-condylar fracture

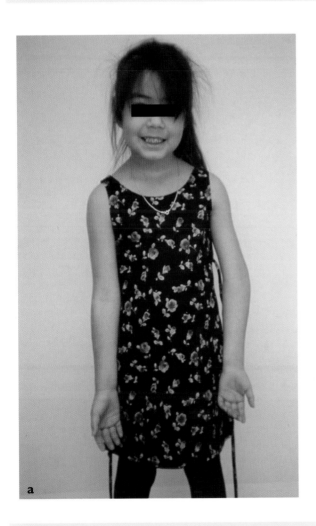
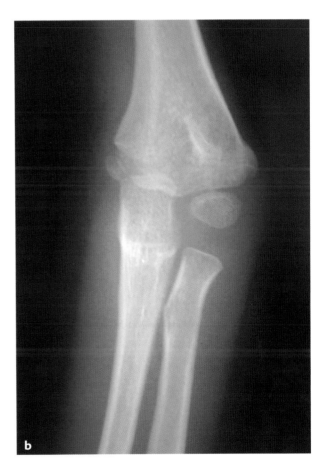

Figure 188 Clinical photograph (a) and anteroposterior radiograph (b) demonstrate the possible late sequelae of angular deformity that can occur if a pediatric elbow fracture is unrecognized or not reduced. Even with proper reduction and fixation, there is a small chance for angulation with any fracture that affects the growth plate

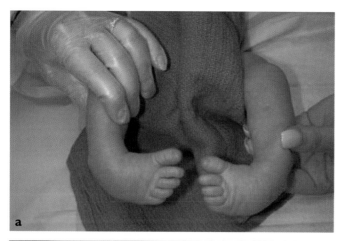

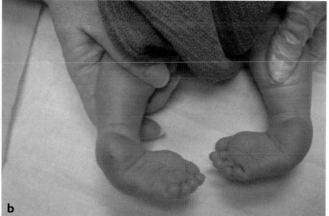

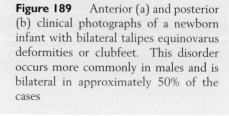

Figure 189 Anterior (a) and posterior (b) clinical photographs of a newborn infant with bilateral talipes equinovarus deformities or clubfeet. This disorder occurs more commonly in males and is bilateral in approximately 50% of the cases

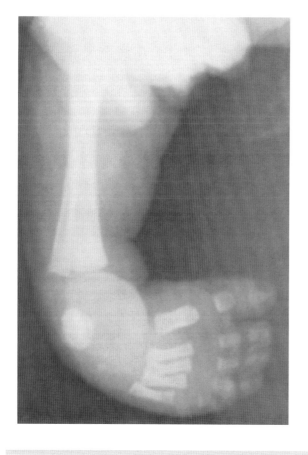

Figure 190 Anteroposterior radiograph of the clubfoot of a newborn; note the varus deformity about the ankle

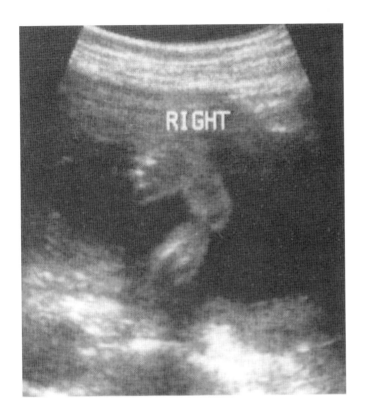

Figure 191 Diagnosis of clubfoot can now be made *in utero* with the use of ultrasound, allowing both the parents and the physicians to formulate and institute a plan of treatment much more rapidly

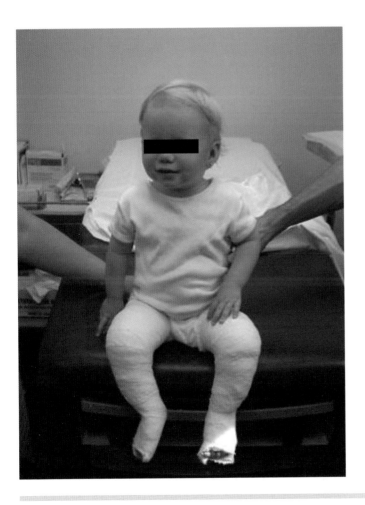

Figure 192 Serial casting is recommended for the first 3–4 months for infants with clubfoot. Much of the time, this serial casting is all that is needed to correct the deformity and allow the children to walk without delay

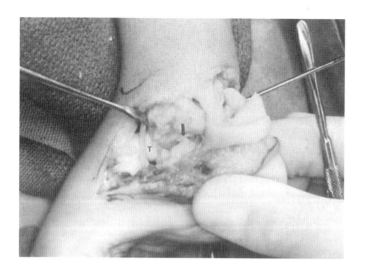

Figure 193 Depending on the severity and age at presentation, surgery for clubfoot has been described with good rates of success

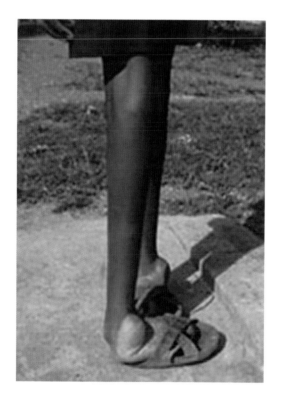

Figure 194 Clinical photograph demonstrating the debilitating natural history of clubbed feet if it is not identified and treated early

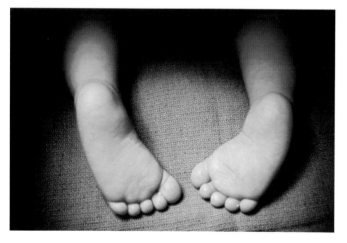

Figure 195 The clinician must be able to distinguish the disorder pictured here, metatarsus adductus, from the more malignant talipes equinovarus. Metatarsus adductus is commonly associated with developmental dysplasia of the hip and generally responds well to stretching, orthotics or casting and rarely requires surgery

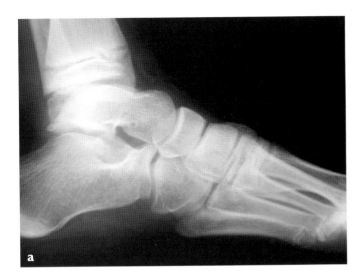

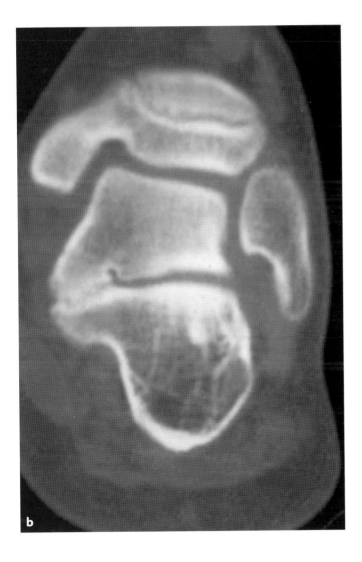

Figure 196 Lateral radiograph (a) and coronal CT scan (b) demonstrating tarsal coalition. This case is a talocalcaneal fusion and the other most common coalition is calcaneonavicular. Patients usually present between the ages of 10 and 12 years with limited motion, flat-foot deformity and calf pain. Tarsal coalition may be fibrous, cartilaginous or osseous. Initial treatment is with immobilization and/or orthotics, but surgery may be required in recalcitrant cases to resect the symptomatic bar

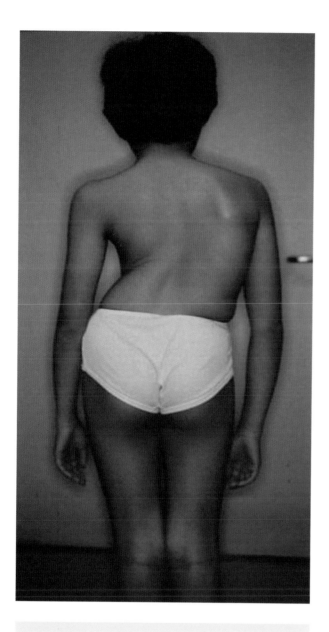

Figure 197 Clinical photograph of a young girl with a severe scoliotic deformity

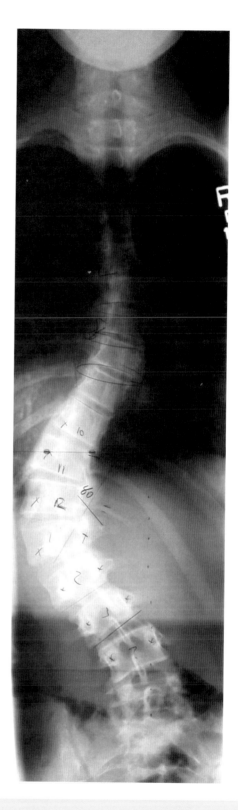

Figure 198 Anteroposterior radiograph of a patient with a right thoracic and left lumbar curve. Most curves that are under 50° can be watched and braced, depending on the level of maturity of the child at presentation. Curves greater than 50° require surgical correction so that the curve does not continue to progress into maturity

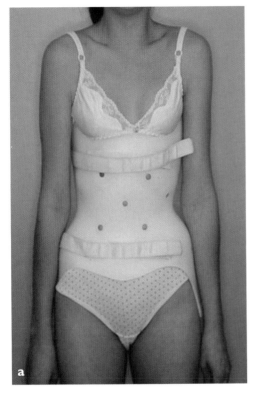

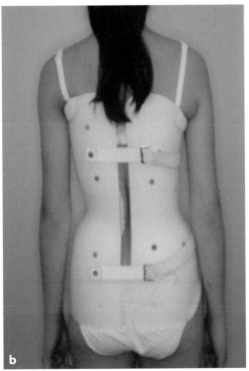

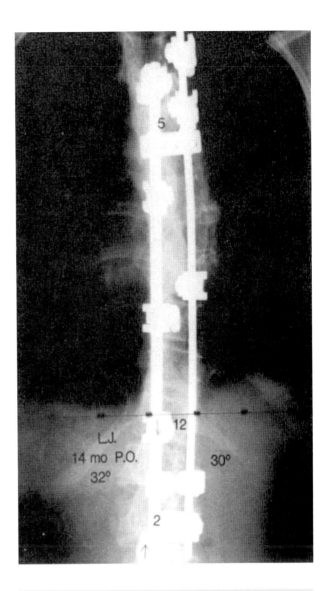

Figure 200 If the scoliotic deformity progresses rapidly or the child is very immature with a larger curve that is likely to progress despite bracing, surgical correction is considered. The curve is corrected using a series of hooks, rods and screws. The most important reason for performing surgery is not the curve correction, but rather the fusion that prevents further advancement of the scoliosis

Figure 199 Photographs illustrating the use of a thoracolumbosacral spinal orthosis (TLSO) brace to slow curve progression while the patient matures. Once the patient matures, the risk of curve progression is very low and the patient can be monitored at longer intervals between radiographs

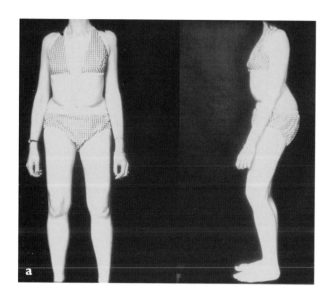

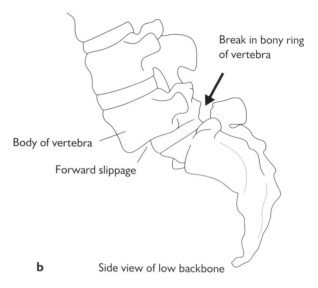

Break in bony ring
of vertebra

Body of vertebra

Forward slippage

b   Side view of low backbone

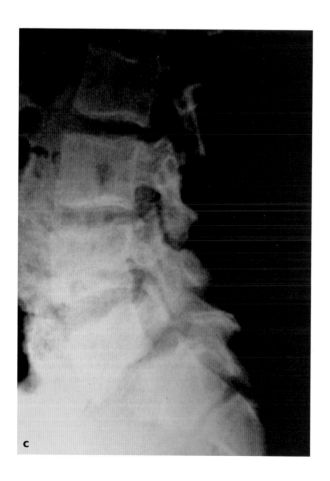

Figure 201   Clinical photographs (a), diagram (b) and lateral radiographs (c) of patients with spondylolisthesis. Spondylolisthesis is a slip of one verte-bra forward on another. The slip occurs due to a defect in the pars intraarticu-laris portion of the spinal ring. The slips are graded based on the percentage of slip – 25%, 50%, etc. In most cases, the slip can be treated with immobilization until it has healed. Rarely, in cases of neural compromise, surgical interven-tion to fuse the slip *in situ* is necessary

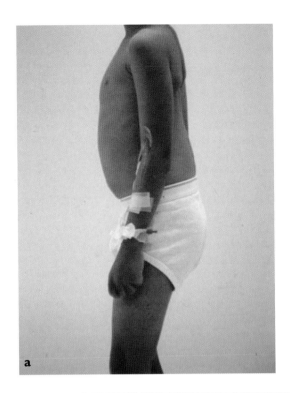
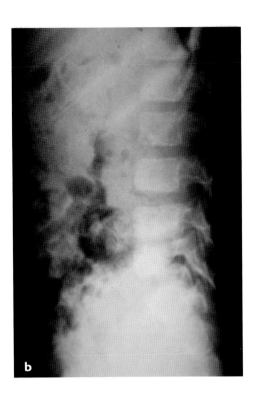

Figures 202 Clinical photograph (a) and lateral radiograph (b) of a young boy with diskitis. Complaints of low back pain should be taken seriously in young children. Diskitis often presents as a refusal by the child to sit or walk and standing with a very rigid flat back posture. The erythrocyte sedimentation rate will be elevated; however, disc space narrowing can often take as long as 3 weeks to show up on plain radiographs. A bone scan is an excellent screening test in the young child with back pain. Diskitis is treated with intravenous antibiotics

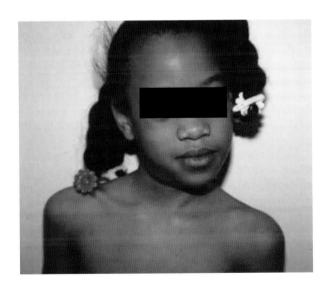
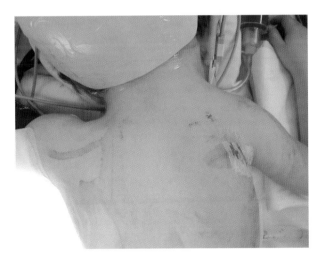

Figure 203 Rotatory atlantoaxial subluxation may present with torticollis, as shown here. It can be caused by retropharyngeal inflammation. Diagnosis is made by CT scan at the C1–C2 junction, with maximal rotation in both directions, and treatment is generally with a combination of traction and bracing. C1–C2 fusion is rarely necessary, in very late presentations

Figure 204 Clinical photo of a patient with Sprengel's deformity on the right, an undescended scapula associated with hypoplasia and winging. It is the most common congenital shoulder abnormality seen in children. Sprengel's deformity is sometimes seen in association with Klippel–Feil syndrome, scoliosis and renal disease

Chapter 8

The spine

Many people are affected by back pain. Every doctor should have an algorithm for addressing back pain so as to recognize the more serious problems. This chapter looks at the cervical, thoracic and lumbar spine and the most common spinal disorders that the clinician encounters.

ANATOMY

Spinal anatomy is generally described by dividing the spine into three major sections: the cervical, the thoracic and the lumbar spine. The area beneath the lumbar spine is called the sacrum and is technically considered to be a part of the pelvis. Each spinal segment is composed of individual vertebral bodies. There are seven cervical vertebrae, 12 thoracic vertebrae and five lumbar vertebrae.

Each vertebra is composed of several parts. The spinous processes are the bones felt when running one's hand down one's back and these project posteriorly. The transverse processes are oriented at right angles to the spinous processes and provide attachment sites for the numerous muscular insertions.

In addition, each vertebra has four facet joints: one pair that face upward and another pair that face downward. These facets connect one vertebra to the next and provide stability to the spine. The bony and ligamentous anatomy of the spine provides a stable structure through which the spinal cord travels. The cord ends between the first and second lumbar vertebrae and continues on as the cauda equina distally. The individual nerve roots exit the spinal canal just beneath their named vertebra (i.e. the C4 nerve root exits just below the fourth cervical vertebra). Injury to the bones or ligaments of the spine can lead to instability which may jeopardize nerve function,

and, thus, must be carefully ruled out in any case of trauma.

The vertebral bodies are separated by cartilaginous discs. These discs function as shock absorbers between the bones. The discs are composed of a tough outer ring called the annulus fibrosis and a more gelatinous center, the nucleus pulposis.

When the disc is injured, the nucleus is able to leak through a tear in the outer annulus. The nucleus can then cause compression and irritation of the surrounding nerve roots, producing symptoms of radicular pain, numbness and/or weakness.

HISTORY AND PHYSICAL EXAMINATION

Pain is often the presenting complaint that brings people in for evaluation. In the spine it is important to determine the location of the pain, and whether the pain is focal or radiating. If the pain is focal, the problem is not likely to involve the spinal cord or nerve roots. However, one must carefully examine and evaluate the upper and/or lower extremities, including a full motor and sensory examination to rule out any nerve or cord involvement.

There are specific provocative tests that one can perform to elicit nerve-related pathology. In the cervical spine, flexion, rotation and compression are used to aggravate radicular symptoms. In the lumbar spine, there are several maneuvers that place tension across the sciatic nerve and, in doing so, further compress an inflamed nerve root against a herniated disc or bone spur. These are termed tension signs. The straight leg raise test is performed with the patient supine. The doctor elevates the leg with the knee kept straight. A positive test occurs when the pain (below the knee) is recreated or exacerbated by this maneuver.

In addition, one must always include an examination of the shoulders and hips when trying to rule out cervical and lumbar pathology, respectively. These areas are frequent sites of referred pain from the spine.

DIAGNOSTIC STUDIES

There are many imaging studies available for use in the spine including plain radiographs, CT scanning, myelography and MRI. Plain radiographs are valuable to rule out conditions such as infection and tumor as well as in the diagnosis of trauma, stenosis, spondylolisthesis and instability. Although radiographs are useful for looking at the bones and alignment, the soft tissues, such as the cord, ligaments and discs, are not visualized. CT scanning and myelography can be helpful in visualizing the soft tissues. MRI is the newest of the diagnostic modalities and, with advancing technology (strength of magnets, surface coils, and pulse sequences), it is rapidly becoming the test of choice for diagnosing spinal pathology.

DISORDERS

Some of the more common spinal disorders are illustrated in Figures 205–220.

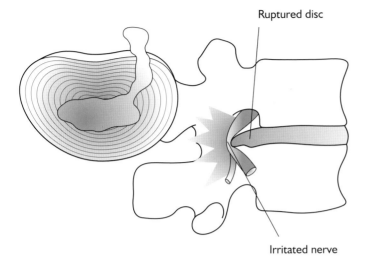

Ruptured disc

Irritated nerve

Figure 205 Diagram of a herniated nucleus pulposus, also called a herniated disc. The disc material generally herniates in a posterolateral direction because of resistance directly posterior from the posterior longitudinal ligament. Acutely herniated discs generally cause radicular pain in the arms (for cervical discs) and down the legs (for lumbar discs); rarely do we see herniated thoracic discs. On physical examination, patients with lumbar herniations will have positive nerve tension signs. With the patient supine, the leg is raised in a straight position. If this maneuver causes recreation of their radicular pain, the test is considered positive

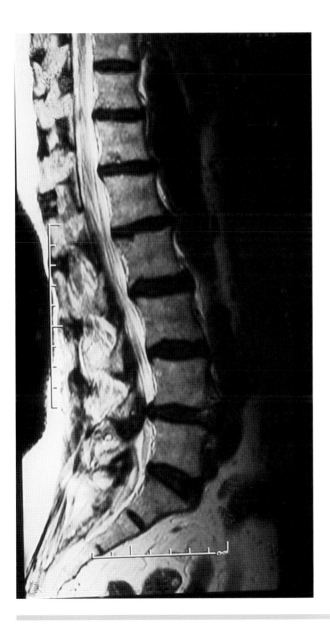

Figure 206 Lateral MRI of a patient with a bulging L4–5 disc. This patient had significant radicular pain that was unresponsive to oral anti-inflammatories and physical therapy. An epidural steroid injection gave this patient significant relief

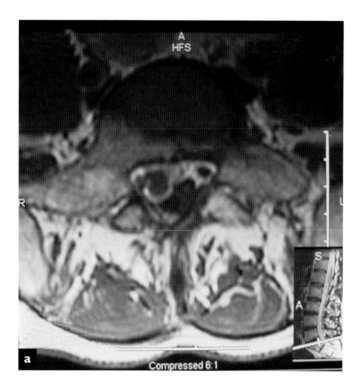

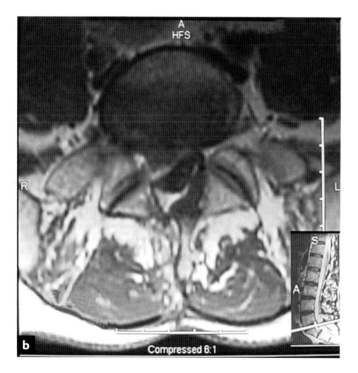

Figures 207 Axial MR images (a) and (b) show a patient with acute onset of pain and motor weakness in his lower extremities. There is a large piece of herniated disc material that is sitting on the right L5 nerve root. The piece is large enough to cause significant compression of the thecal sac (the spinal cord itself ends proximally at the L2 level) and nerve roots. This patient underwent surgical excision of the disc. The motor loss resolved and his pain was relieved soon after surgery

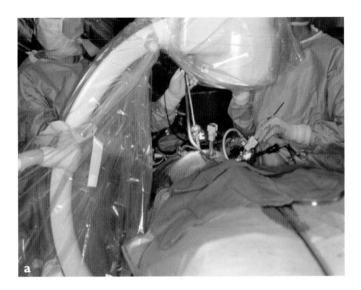

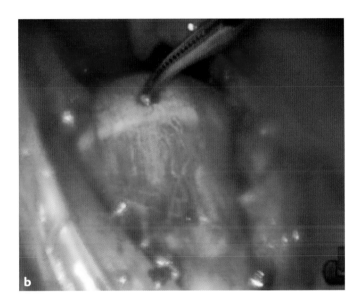

Figure 208 Newer techniques of spinal surgery include endoscopic decompressions. The operating room set-up is shown in (a) as well as the endoscopic photograph of disc localization (b) and removal (c)

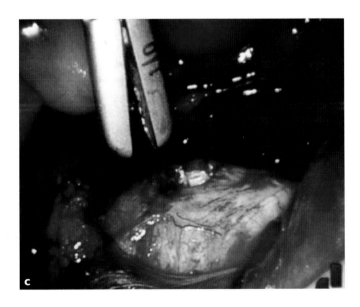

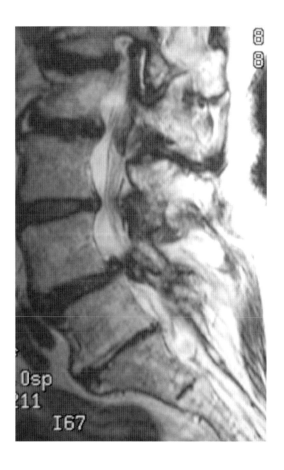

Figure 209 Lateral MRI demonstrating significant lumbar spinal stenosis. Patients with lumbar spinal stenosis often complain of pain and numbness in their legs with prolonged standing or walking. The pain tends to resolve when the patient leans forward (relieving the pressure on the nerves) or sits down. The excess bone impinges on the nerve roots as they exit the foramen causing the radicular symptoms

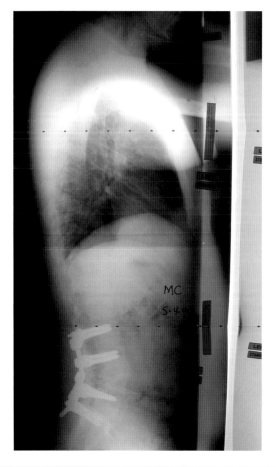

Figure 210 For some patients with early stenosis, epidural steroid injection will help. If the radicular symptoms persist, patients may undergo a surgical decompression of the nerve and, in some cases (depending on the amount of bone removed), a fusion with instrumentation is necessary to stabilize the spine. This is a lateral radiograph of a patient who underwent a decompression and fusion for spinal stenosis

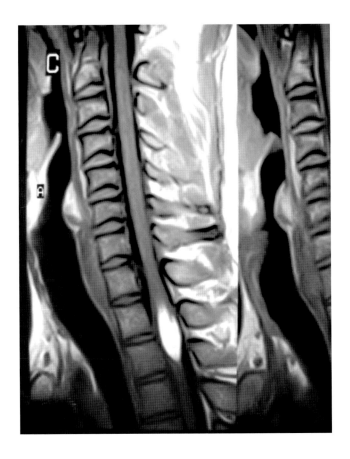

Figure 211 Lateral MRI demonstrating a spinal cord tumor. Spinal cord tumors are very rare and difficult to treat

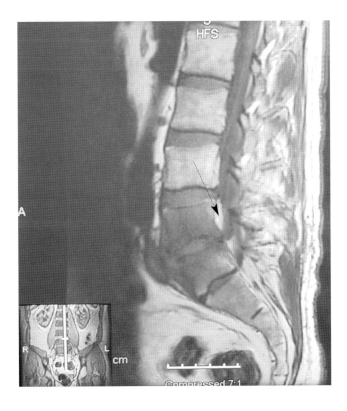

Figure 212 A patient with a spinal infection. The sagittal MRI clearly shows disc space involvement as well as involvement of L4 and L5. Note the decreased signal in those vertebral bodies. Just posterior to the L4–5 disc is a small collection of fluid indicating an epidural abscess

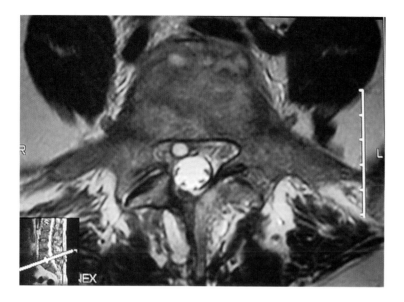

Figure 213   Axial MRI of the same patient as in Figure 212 with the abscess seen clearly in the epidural space. This patient underwent irrigation and debridement and long-term treatment with intravenous antibiotics

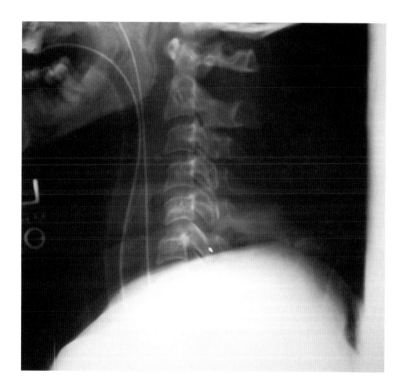

Figure 214   Lateral radiograph of the cervical spine. In addition to the C5–6 subluxation that is apparent on this radiograph, it is important to realize that, in most lateral radiographs of the cervical spine, the last cervical vertebra is not visualized due to a shadow from the chest and shoulders. It is very important in the emergency setting, when trying to rule out trauma, to obtain a clear picture of the entire cervical spine to C7. This can be difficult due to a patient's body habitus and CT scanning is often necessary

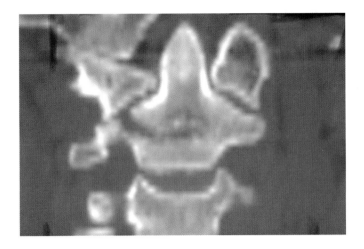

Figure 215 CT scan showing a fracture at the base of the dens process. These fractures are often difficult to see on plain radiographs. If there is any question, a CT scan is very useful

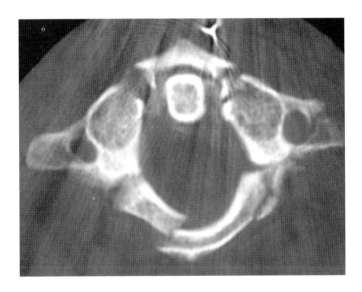

Figure 216 Axial CT scan illustrating a burst fracture of the ring of C1, called a Jefferson burst fracture. These fractures are often unstable, and must be carefully evaluated with the help of CT to determine the plan of treatment. Most often, these fractures are reduced and treated with halo traction. C1–2 fusion is indicated in cases of non-union

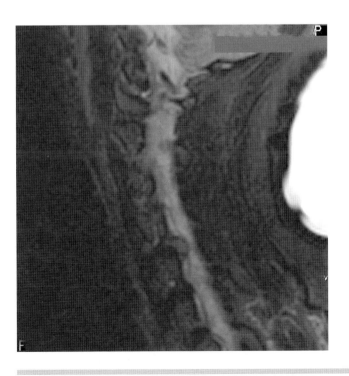

Figure 217 Sagittal MRI demonstrating a herniated cervical disc. Herniations in the cervical spine cause radicular symptoms in the upper extremities. Herniated cervical discs are treated similarly to those in the lumbar spine. Physical therapy, oral anti-inflammatories, and steroid injections are often helpful. For those cases that fail conservative treatment or have significant associated weakness, surgical excision of the herniated disc is recommended to alleviate their symptoms

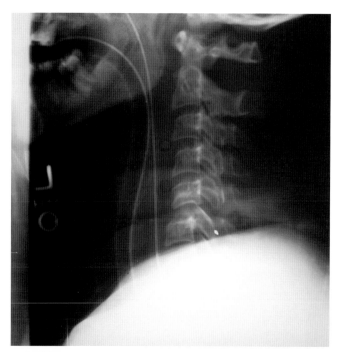

Figure 218 Lateral radiograph of a patient with C5–6 instability. This patient has only mild degenerative changes, but instability is often associated with degenerative disc disease

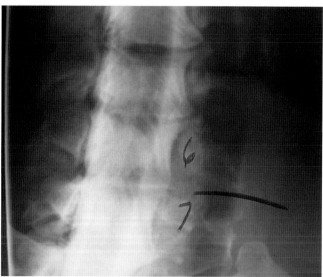

Figure 219 A cervical myelogram is shown here. This is a very useful test to visualize any impedence to the spinal cord. The myelogram will demonstrate a filling defect if there is either bony or soft tissue blocking the path of the cord

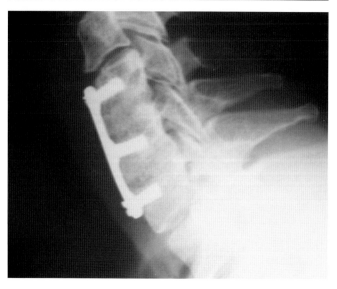

Figure 220 A lateral radiograph of a patient who underwent an anterior cervical fusion for instability and degenerative disease. Cervical decompressions and fusions can be approached from both the front (as seen here) or the back (a posterior approach). Most cervical pathology can be addressed through both approaches. Diagnosis as well as surgeon preference generally dictate the approach used. The anterior approach is a muscle-splitting approach and, since there is little tissue dissection, the recovery is faster

Bibliography

1. Rockwood CA, Green DP, Bucholz RW, Heckman JD, eds. *Fractures in Adults*, 4th edn. Philadelphia: Lippincott-Raven, 1996

2. Rockwood CA, Wilkins KE, Beaty JH. *Fractures in Children*, 4th edn. Philadelphia: Lippincott-Raven, 1996

3. Canale ST, ed. *Campbell's Operative Orthopaedics*, 9th edn. St. Louis: Mosby-Year Book, 1998

4. McGinty JB, Caspari RB, Jackson RW, Poehling GG, eds. *Operative Arthroscopy*, 2nd edn. Philadelphia: Lippincott-Raven, 1996

5. Rockwood CA, Matsen III FA, eds. *The Shoulder*, 2nd edn. Philadelphia: WB Saunders, 1998

6. Wiesel SW, Delahay JN, Connell MC, eds. *Essentials of Orthopaedic Surgery*. Philadelphia: WB Saunders, 1993

7. Beaty JH, ed. *Orthopaedic Knowledge Update 6: Home Study Syllabus*. Rosemont, IL: American Academy of Orthopedic Surgeons, 1999

8. Miller MD, ed. *Review of Orthopedics*, 3rd edn. Philadelphia: WB Saunders, 2000

Index